Running My Loop

31 Days of Unfiltered Thoughts and Observations While Pushing Myself for a Half-Marathon PR

by

Manley Peterson

Dedicated to runners everywhere. And of every shape. Sometimes, I'm a circle.

BACKSTORY: I started running in 2013 because my lower back hurt. I sat too much and didn't exercise enough. My desk job pretty much guaranteed bad posture, poor health, and aches and pains. I thought of myself as athletic and in good shape, but when I looked at my body in the mirror, I wasn't happy with my visibly plump waist and belly fat. Also, a check-up at the doctor noted my cholesterol and blood pressure were too high. If I wanted a healthier, longer life, it was time for me to exercise more. I decided to try running, since I didn't really need anything more than comfortable shoes, a GPS watch, and a safe area to run around.

In 2013, I ran a total of 42 times for 170 miles, but I didn't know what I was doing. In 2014, I ran 106 times for 408 miles, but I was injured all the time. In 2015, I ran 63 times for 217 miles, but I wasn't disciplined enough to run more. In 2016, I ran 153 times for 573 miles. That was the first year I was determined to make progress and beat my PRs. I forced myself to get outside and run, even in the snow, ice, heat, and rain.

I am not a professional runner. I have not been trained by anyone. I am not sponsored by a company. I am not paid to run. I am not in great shape. I am just a normal middle-aged man. I have a normal day job with a normal work week. I have a normal family and normal life. For all intents and purposes, I am just like you.

But winter months are hard on my body. The weather is awful and many days are not runnable in rural Wisconsin due to extreme cold or ice or snowfall. By the end of December 2016, I was miserable and feeling bad about my physical condition. I wanted to get outside and do something—anything. Run, walk, whatever. But most days the weather would not cooperate. As the cold, winter days dragged on, I decided to make a goal for New Year's 2017. I would plan to accumulate 720 miles in one year. I would need to average 60 miles per month or 2 miles per day. I knew that the winter months would be against me, so I planned to ramp up the miles when the sun was shining in the summer months.

Here is what I have accomplished so far:

Month	Runs	Mileage	Total/Goal	Progress
January	6	30.32	30.32/60	-29.68
February	9	30.05	60.37/120	-59.63
March	14	40.83	101.20/180	-78.80
April	14	60.13	161.33/240	-78.67
May	30	100.61	261.94/300	-38.06
June	30	128.97	390.91/360	+30.91

It took a full six months, but I was finally able to break even and then get ahead of my monthly goals.

And that brings me to July 2017. The following pages are basically a daily journal of my unfiltered thoughts and observations as I continued running trying to better myself. Each day was written out the same day I ran. Sometimes I had enough time to write immediately after the run. Sometimes I had to wait until the end of the day to write, because I needed to jet off to work immediately after running. So, you will see a jumble of thoughts and feelings. You will see good days and bad days. Sometimes I wrote in the present tense, sometimes I wrote in the past tense. You will see short phrases that barely meet the requirements to be a sentence. And you will read run-on sentences and wonder when it will stop. And you might see paragraphs longer than single pages and single pages shorter than paragraphs. I think it is all readable, and I'm not going to change any of it. I'm not trying to win a literature prize. This book is what I was at each point in my monthly journey. I want you to remember that the journey is just as important as the destination.

Saturday, July 1 from 7:20 AM to 8:10 AM

Splits	Time	Cumulative Time	Distance
1	8:52.8	08:52	1.00
2	8:44.2	17:37	1.00
3	8:57.2	26:34	1.00
4	8:52.7	35:27	1.00
5	9:00.3	44:27	1.00
6	5:34.0	50:01	0.65
Summary	50:01	50:01	5.65 mi
Average Pace 8:51 min/mi			

PRE-RUN: I got up around 6:30 AM and felt okay. I had a single cup of coffee. I had about four pieces of pizza the night before and a single can of soda. I felt pretty good in morning, did some stretches. I had just finished a full month of running at least 4 miles every day. I thought about what kind of goal I should set for July. I settled upon running enough each day to accumulate 24 hours by the end of July, so that I could say that I ran for what amounts to one whole day in a single month. I got dressed in my Brooks Ghost 9 shoes, white socks, Batman pajama pants, a cotton t-shirt, a black running hood with face muffler, and a baseball cap. Looking outside, it didn't seem too hot or sunny, but I put sunscreen on my face and arms anyway, anticipating I would need to open the face part of the hood eventually. I used my Garmin Forerunner 10 GPS watch for timing.

RUNNING: Once outside, the temperature seemed good with a little bit of wind. I decided upon a nice easy run to get a good baseline for the rest of the month. I started to sing Patrick Swayze's song "She's Like the Wind." I can butcher about two lines, and then it is repeat, repeat, repeat. I tried to do the math in my head and settled upon 45 minutes running every day with a half-marathon on last day to try for a new record. My half-marathon record at the time was 1h 56m 1s, which is 8:51 min/mile pace. I figured if I could stay around 9 minutes per mile for this whole month, my body would be ready to run the half and break my record. As I was running, I noticed lots of ant hills on the loop. No neighbors were out. No neighborhood pets were out. A stupid deer fly (or maybe a horse fly) bit me on the back of my neck right below the hood fabric. Also, I got an eyelash or small bug in my right eye for a few agonizing seconds, but it fixed itself. It wasn't super humid, but bad enough that my shirt was half soaked, and it made wiping my face and nose unpleasant. I think somewhere around the third mile, I started to do the math again on my 24-hour time goal and realized that 45 minutes per day would not be enough. It would take 32 days to get to 24 hours at 45 minutes per day. I decided to just do 50 minutes a day and anything over 24 hours would be fine. *Just a fool to believe, she's like the wind.* As I ran, the clouds stayed out and didn't move much. I hardly saw the sun at all, although the few times I looked up, the sky was still too bright even with the cloud cover. At one point, I ran over a dead earthworm. I didn't run on him, but just passed over him. He was completely pale, and I think the local ants were taking care of him, but it was tough to focus on a small thing like that when running by. It must have rained the previous night, because the gravel and sand and pebbles were sticking to my shoes. They would kick up and hit my pant legs and slowly and surely get into my socks and shoes. It wasn't horrible. I've had worse days, but any kind of rock or sand in my shoes makes me unhappy. I ended up with 5.65 miles after 50 minutes with an 8:51 pace. When 50 minutes had passed, I stopped running and walked to my blacktop driveway for stretching. I didn't feel tired or worn out while running. I thought this pace felt good and was confident I could keep this up for more miles. I thought this was a good start. I did bend over waist stretches to my toes and one squat and then some quick yoga stretches for my back, then lay on my belly for two quad stretches. While lying face down, flies buzzed all around my head. One landed on my nose and wouldn't move until I swatted it away. As I walked back in the house, a deer fly bit me in the left shoulder. Was that Mother Nature's parting blow? Get out of here Manley and go back to your home.

POST-RUN: I did the math again, but this time on paper instead of my head. I found out that running 50 minutes a day will get me to 24 hours on day 29. That will be 2 days ahead of schedule. If my math is right, the end of the 31st day will equal 25 hours, 50 minutes of running. Now I realize that 45 minutes was the right amount to begin with, ha-ha! On day 30, my total time at 45 minutes per day is 22 hours and 30 minutes. And then when I run my half-marathon on day 31, it should take me over 1 hour and 30 minutes (but hopefully under my record of 1 hour, 56 minutes), so that would get me to just over my 24-hour goal. So, I guess I ran an extra 5 minutes today for no reason. I'll consider it a little padding. My weight after a shower was 168.2 pounds.

Sunday, July 2 from 8:19 AM to 9:09 AM

Splits	Time	Cumulative Time	Distance
1	8:37.1	08:37	1.00
2	8:25.3	17:02	1.00
3	8:38.6	25:41	1.00
4	8:35.1	34:16	1.00
5	8:43.6	43:00	1.00
6	7:01.5	50:01	0.80
Summary	50:01	50:01	5.80 mi
Average Pace 8:37 min/mi			

PRE-RUN: I got up around 7:17 AM and had a slight headache, so I drank a coffee to perk up. I noticed it was all sunny outside. I did my stretches. I also sucked in huge amounts of air, pretending my chest was a big balloon. I did that probably five times. In my mind, I was saturating my cells with oxygen so they perform better. It might just be a mental thing. I got dressed in Brooks Ghost 9 shoes, white socks, green money-print pajama pants, blue cotton t-shirt, no hood today, and baseball cap. Last night I attended a wedding and pigged out on six large cups of root beer and huge amounts of Chex Mix, along with the full meal of chicken, potatoes, corn, and beans. I was a little worried all that food would affect my running today, but (as usual) I didn't stop eating it anyway.

RUNNING: Okay, I ran 50 minutes yesterday. That wasn't the plan. The plan was 45 minutes, and now I was thinking that it would be silly to go back to only doing 45-minute runs again. It would just feel wrong to me. So, I guess an extra 5 minutes a day won't kill me. It'll put me way over my 24-hour goal, but I guess I do that with my goals. I always seem to set a goal, and then immediately try to destroy it by going above and beyond. I'm not sure why I do that. Why don't I just set the higher goal to begin with? So, anyway, I guess I'm all in at the 50 minutes per day now. It also has the built-in bonus of an attempt at breaking my 10K record every single day. My record was 49 minutes, 4 seconds, so if I am forcing myself to run 50 minutes a day, there is always a chance I'll have a great day and break the 10K record. I'm not going to consciously try for it, but if after the first mile or two I am at a good record pace, I might try it then. Patrick Swayze was back. *She's like the wind. Just a fool to believe. I don't know the words, just a foooool to believe. She's like the wind.* There aren't any bugs out here. That's a relief. I hate it when they buzz around. I've literally had multiple flies pester me for miles around the loop. They flit around, land on my hat or my face or my neck, and then I'm either forced to swat them away or they fly away on their own after sucking up my precious sweat. But they never ever leave for long. They don't go far. But today, no bugs. I did hear them in the weeds as I ran by, though. Plenty of background noise of buzzing and chirping. My own personal orchestra. Birds too, singing or cheeping or chirping, and then moving in the tall grass and brush. Big crows were high up in the trees, cawing to each other. Today was really a perfect weather day. My body felt strong. I settled into a good rhythm. I really think a 9 minute per mile pace is my natural pace. It feels normal and easy. If I go slower, it is tougher on my body. The slowdown feels wrong. If I go faster, it is tougher on my body. The speedup feels wrong. To speed up or slow down takes mental energy and mental focus. At the 9 minute pace, I don't have to think. My body is on auto-pilot. I just move. My strides feel the right length. I'm also glad I put on lots of sunscreen and went without my black hood. I feel less constricted. And I think I can cool down better during the run. When that black hood gets soaking wet, it kinda feels like a heavy wet blanket around my neck and head. I usually choose to wear it during cold weather, but today, I'm glad I went without it. Around my gravel loop, I noticed all the little craters below my feet. Millions of them. It rained hard last night for about 20 minutes, could have been longer, but I remember waking up when the downpour happened. It browbeat the gravel loop into submission. Millions of little divots, craters, pockmarks. The loop looked new and different. And now my shoe prints were clearly visible as I ran around the loop and turned back on my previous paths. Single paths become many paths and dozens and dozens of footfalls become hundreds of steps. I'd done the math in my head while running the loop before, if each of my strides is roughly 3 feet, then a single mile is about 1,700 steps. So, on longer runs, like a 10-miler or more, it is amazing to think I've taken 17,000 steps or even 20,000 steps in a single run. Anyway, that's not happening today. Focus on this 50-minute run on this fresh gravel loop. It isn't hard for me to imagine I'm taking the first human steps on a virgin landscape, perhaps on another world. The gray dust of the loop looked like our moon sometimes. Perhaps I'm the first human on this terrain. Maybe the first person to sing here, too? *Just a fool to believe, she's like the wind. She's like the wind.* I checked my watch a few times. I can tell my pace was faster than yesterday, which is expected because the weather is nice; I felt good. And I've finally decided on just doing the 50 minutes per day. My watch beeps every mile and gives me my mile pace. I can see I'm running under 9 minutes per mile, about 20 to 30 seconds faster. Still, to beat my 10K record, I would need to be much faster. About 7:50 minutes per mile, but I'm not going to get close to that today. That isn't my plan. The sun is strong. No clouds. The heat is not bad, but the warmth is all over my body. Sometimes I imagine myself as Superman. Sucking in all that yellow sun energy and stoking my fire, giving me strength to excel at running. I think of that Seinfeld episode where Jerry and George are discussing if the yellow sun augments all of Superman's powers, then Superman must have a super sense of humor. Jerry can't wrap his head around why the yellow sun would give Superman super speed and strength, but not humor. George ends it with something like "Well, all I know is, he ain't funny." Even with the perfect weather, I'm still sweating. It is always my face that I am wiping. My legs get sweaty, also my back and chest and arms and neck, but those don't bother me. It is always my face and nose and brow. A couple swipes of my t-shirt across my nose produces a squeaky noise. It sounds like a mouse or maybe a dog's chew toy. It is funny sometimes, but mostly the sweat just smears. My soaked shirt can no longer do anything. It is saturated. Again, back to the weather. I realize that if today is perfect, that means it can only go downhill from here. I'm on day 2. That means the next 29 days will only be this or worse. Probably much worse. There will be cloudy days, humid days, rainy and stormy days. There will be days that I will need to run later in the day instead of early morning, due to work or bad weather or other commitments, so my body will be full of food or aches or exhaustion. That kinda depresses me. In northern Wisconsin, there are basically only three good running months. Besides, June, July, and August, it is nothing but snow or wind or rain or storms or cold, cold, cold. I need to soak this day up. File it away in my memory and remember it when I need to. For when I'm running during a bad day. I finish the 50 minutes with 5.80 miles. That is .15 more than yesterday. That is good. And when I stop running, I am not breathing hard. I can easily stand there and slowly take deep breaths and walk to my driveway for post stretching. This was definitely a good run day.

POST-RUN: During my bend at the waist stretching, two vertebrate bones pulled away from each other in my lower back. It feels like air rushing into the voids. My backbone must get compressed while running for so long. My hamstrings get tight after runs. Overall, I felt good. I think I was on a runner's high. I feel high confidence for the rest of the day. The weather was gorgeous and that plays a huge part in my good mood. I'm lying face down on my blacktop stretching my quads. I turn my head to the left or right, which is opposite the leg I'm stretching. The sun is on my face when I look left. *I'm just a fool to believe, the sun's like the wind. Oh, that sun feels good, she's like the wind.* Oh Patrick, I can't explain why my mind does that. I apologize for the bad song lyrics, but you'll just have to deal with it. My weight after a shower was 165.7 pounds (down 2.5).

Monday, July 3 from 6:29 AM to 7:19 AM

Splits	Time	Cumulative Time	Distance
1	8:36.4	08:36	1.00
2	8:34.9	17:11	1.00
3	8:41.3	25:53	1.00
4	8:56.9	34:49	1.00
5	9:04.9	43:54	1.00
6	6:06.1	50:00	0.70
Summary	50:00	50:00	5.70 mi
Average Pace 8:47 min/mi			

PRE-RUN: I woke up at 5:30 AM today, because I needed to get my morning routine and running done in time to get to work by 8:00 AM. I figured if I could be out running no later than 6:30 AM, then I would be done by 7:20 and have enough time to shower and change and leave for work. I noticed my lower back ached. I tried to stretch it out, but it didn't help much. It cracked a little. I got dressed in Brooks Ghost 9 shoes, white socks, green ninja turtle pajama pants, blue cotton t-shirt, black hood, and baseball cap. It seemed sunny and warm outside, but the temperature on my phone said it was 51 degrees, so I decided to wear the hood. I never know if that is a good thing or bad thing, since the hood gives sun protection and warmth, but after a while it can become a damp nuisance. I had one cup of coffee.

RUNNING: My back worried me a little, but in past runs, the circulation and warming up usually made my back feel better. Patrick Swayze is taking a break. But my earworm (getting a specific song or song lyric stuck in your head) is now in full effect. Now, I'm singing Steppenwolf's "Born to be Wild." *Hit the motor running, heading for the highway, looking for adventure, yeah, whatever comes my way.* And that magically morphs into Silverchair's "Freak." *Yeah, I'm a freak...of nature. I don't really know. How to put on a good show. Boring as they come...* Good ole Silverchair. Haven't listened to that band in a long time, not sure how that got into my head. Sometime in the first mile or two, I had a coffee burp, and it went right into my black hood muffler. That was pretty disgusting. This is one of the reasons I always brush my teeth before running, because sometimes the most putrid and awful smelling things come out of your mouth when you are working hard. After my good run yesterday and distance improvement, I reminded myself that I didn't need to be Superman every day. I just needed to be Manley today. And whatever happens, happens. The first two miles felt good, and with split times in the 8:30 mile range, I figured I would have another good day. But then, at the beginning of mile three, I felt my left hip start twinging and pulling and generally yelling at me. I did some butt kicks and high knees to try to stretch it out while still running. I think they might have helped a bit, but from that point on, I could just tell this wasn't going to be my day. And that was proved truth by my split times for miles three, four, and five getting progressively slower. Running by some tall grass, I heard an animal noise. I looked down a side road and hoped it wasn't a bear. Luckily, just a mother turkey and two cute little babies. Upon seeing or hearing me, she took off running with babies in tow. It is kinda funny, as I run around that loop, I hear animals in the tall grass but cannot see them. Then, when I'm close enough and whatever it is gets frightened, I hear a movement or a crashing in the brush. I rarely see the culprit, though. When I do, it is usually a bird flying away into a tree, but other times it has been a rabbit. I can deal with those, but I'm not sure what I could do if it was a big carnivore. I imagine it wouldn't feel good to be surprised like that. Fight or flight response. I try to picture my heart like a strong cannon, shooting out blood to my entire body. Maybe like that spread shot gun from *Contra* on NES? Yesterday, my gravel loop was like an alien landscape with all those little craters in the sand and dirt. Today, that is all gone and replaced with tire tracks round and round the loop from neighbors and other traffic. I think it would be cool if I could see all the past "me" ghosts running around the loop like in *Super Mario Kart* on SNES. I could race against myself. I kept the black hood muffler on for the first two miles, but had to take it off. It was getting too hot and sweaty. With it on, it is like I'm a fireplace bellows. The fabric fills out with my breathing out, and then gets sucked back in as I breathe in. The fabric sticks to my face for split seconds. I don't really care for that, but I put it out of my mind. I see the neighbor's dog is out by his garage. The dog just looks at me. Most times in the past, he has barked at me. But today he is silent. I don't know why he barks some days and not others. Maybe he is enjoying the quiet time outside, too. And he doesn't want to mar it with a vulgar bark. Suddenly, I realize that July 31st might not be a weekend. I am going to run my half-marathon on the 31st. What day is that? July 1st was a Saturday, so July 8th, 15th, 22nd. Oh no, 29th is a Saturday. That means the 31st is a Monday. Argh. That is a work day! Not what I want. Now I will have to take the morning off from work. No way do I want to try to run that half really early in morning and get to work on time. Oh, well, it has to be done. This is important to me. I like having these goals. Miles 4 and 5 take longer than I'm used to compared with the last few days. Only about 20 to 30 seconds longer, but it is noticeable. I am keeping my arms close to my body and as they swing out in front of me, I pretend I am throwing body blows at the world or air or whatever. It takes my mind off my hip pain. I feel like Little Mac in *Mike Tyson's Punch-out* on NES. That's the third video game reference, I must want to play something. There, I look at my watch in time to see the 50 minutes passed, and I press stop on my Garmin. My watch will only beep at the splits, so I hear it at miles 1, 2, 3, etc. But due to my roughly 9 minutes per mile pace and running for 50 minutes, I won't get a nice beep at the cut-off time. I have to pay attention and make sure I stop my watch at 50 minutes, so as that last minute counts down, I find myself glancing at the watch every few seconds. I start walking to my driveway for cool-down stretches.

POST-RUN: I notice I'm not breathing hard. Is that good or bad? I immediately think it is good. I must be in good cardiovascular shape, right? That kinda makes me feel good about myself. Or is it bad? Maybe I'm not pushing myself hard enough. I know my pace isn't crazy, but running for 50 minutes every single day, and so far, going over 5.5 miles per day, that seems pretty good. When I started running four years ago, there is no way I could have run straight for 50 minutes without breathing hard. If, and that is a big if, I could have finished 50 minutes back then, I would have been sucking air so hard, I might have fallen over from hyperventilation. But today, I feel good. I mean, other than my left hip, I feel good. I decide that not breathing heavy is a good thing. Good job, Manley. My weight after a shower was 166.6 pounds (up 0.9).

Tuesday, July 4 from 7:09 AM to 7:59 AM

Splits	Time	Cumulative Time	Distance
1	8:44.9	08:44	1.00
2	8:31.2	17:16	1.00
3	8:40.4	25:56	1.00
4	8:35.7	34:32	1.00
5	8:35.8	43:08	1.00
6	6:53.2	50:01	0.80
Summary	50:01	50:01	5.80 mi
Average Pace 8:37 min/mi			

PRE-RUN: I woke up for the day around 6:00 AM, but it was a restless sleep all night. My neighbors came home around 2:00 AM from wherever and revved their truck engine. And their night wouldn't be complete unless there was screaming and yelling about something, a few f-bombs dropped, and their house door slammed. This doesn't happen often, but once a week is enough for me. Other than that annoyance, I just think I was anxious for my next run to see what I could do. My injuries from the previous day were on my mind. How would my left hip respond? Getting out of bed brought more bad news. My right knee, right in front, had a sharp pain. Not sure where that came from. I did my regular morning stretches and had one cup of coffee. I didn't wear the black hood today. Just Ghost 9 shoes, white socks, blue shorts, and gray shirt with ball cap. I lathered up my face and arms and legs in sunscreen, and remembered my arm pits were feeling sore. I decided to lube up a few chafed spots with petroleum jelly. I have been running for a while, so I don't think this is normal chafing from two parts rubbing together. I am blaming this on my new deodorant. I think it is irritating my skin there, so I've switched to another kind to see what happens. I'm off work today because of the Fourth of July holiday, so that allows me to relax. Less stress with not having to feel like I gotta rush and get to work.

RUNNING: I started running gingerly, waiting to see what happened with my left hip. Would it be okay? Would it suddenly flare up and explode? And my right knee, what was going on with that? I took the first mile at a normal pace and was pleasantly surprised it was an 8:44 pace and my legs felt good. Maybe they just needed to work themselves out? I'm also helping myself by running in the middle of the road around the loop. This is a township gravel road, so it is rounded to help with water run-off. This means the middle of the road is the top of a dome and as it goes out to the sides, it starts to decline. Ever so slightly you are running with one leg shorter than the other. Usually, I do run the outside of the loop, but I figure it comes out in a wash because I always retrace my steps so my left and right legs are getting equal length. But today I would just do the middle. *And I'm moving right along. Fancy free. Dum-de-de-dum, dum-de-de-dum. Moving right along.* Kermit the Frog and

Fozzie Bear's "Movin' Right Along" driving song popped into my head. Mostly appropriate for running, I guess. Nature was calling. I always go to the bathroom before running, but the coffee must have been fast-acting today. I probably could've held my pee, but I still had over 40 minutes left to run, and I didn't want to think about it anymore. I decide to run down Pee Lane and get it over with. I call this little off-shoot road Pee Lane, because I've used it a few times just for this very reason. The road goes nowhere, just ends at a farmer's field. It was meant to connect to another loop, if the housing development ever took off here, but with the housing bubble burst, it never happened. I paused my running watch, did my business, and in less than 20 seconds, I'd restarted my watch, and continued on this run. Little did I know that I'd acquired two stowaways. More on that in mile three. I ran past my back yard and there were six large crows walking around back there. Looking for worms or whatever they can find, I'm guessing. Man, they get big. I called them big black chickens, because I'm pretty sure they rival that size. Sometimes they are quiet, but today they were caw-caw-cawing away at each other. I watched a show that said crows are super smart and can differentiate between people and locations. I wonder what they say about me? During the first mile, I heard the far neighbor's big dog bark twice and then just silence. I'm guessing that my neighbor took his dog inside, because I didn't hear it bark again during the entire run. This gravel loop is pretty beat-up I noticed. There are 4-wheeler tracks everywhere, again from one of my other neighbor's family. Some of the ruts are annoying, and I wished they weren't there. For a loop with only four houses on it, this road sure gets a lot of extra traffic. As I made my turn at the end of my road, which intersects a major state highway, I saw a lone bicyclist heading south. He was wearing a bright yellow safety jacket and helmet. I waved to the biker and he waved back. I thought it was a guy, but I couldn't be 100% sure. I wonder if that could be a future me? Perhaps I got older and my knees gave out, so I had to bike for exercise. The biker went right on by, wheeling away past my road. Only he knows where to. Maybe he couldn't stop since he is from the future, and he is worried about paradoxes and time discrepancies and horrible things like that. I respected that time-traveling biker more and more with each step. Especially if he really is me from the future. Go Future Manley, go. Now the other neighbor's dog was out. This one usually barks, but stays close to his garage and doesn't chase me. I appreciate that. I don't want to be eaten by man's best friend. But today, he just watches as I run by. Still, I move away from the center of the road and run on the other edge in the sparse grass. I want to give a big enough space to assure the dog I'm safe. I wonder what he thinks. His head turns slowly as he tracks me for many steps. Does he think I'm food? Maybe not fast food, but middle-aged "trying to be in good shape" food? I notice an animal landmine just in time to sidestep it. Out here in the Northwoods, there are lots of animals. And where there are lots of animals, there are landmines. Otherwise known as poop piles. This one is a beautiful shade of dark green, about the size of a golf ball, and glistening in the morning sun. It is like poop poetry. I have no idea what animal left that there for me to find. But I file it away in my head so I will not step in it on my return trips around the loop. My son said a funny thing yesterday. We had seen a green frog near our pond, and he got out his animal identification book to figure out what it was. He decided it was the American Green Frog (yes, I know, how did they come up with such a descriptive name?). And then he laughed and said, "I wonder if the animals do the same thing when we leave? Like, did that frog hop over to his frog family and get out their human identification book, and say, "I don't know what those things were, but we'll see if we can find them in here. Ah yes, here it is. The American human. Mostly fat and stupid." *Moving right along, fancy free, I'm moving, just you and me. Moving right along.* At mile 3.5, I get a sharp twinge in the back of my right knee. Oh, so now it starts. This will balloon into a huge injury, and I'll never finish my monthly goal, much less this run today. But about five steps later, the pain was gone and didn't come back. But then I notice that my upper back feels peculiar. Small little stings. I keep running but look over my right shoulder. There is a big deer fly sucking my soul dry. I swat him away the best I can, and figure I better look to my left. And of course, because why not, there is a deer fly on my left shoulder giving me the business. I swat that one away, too. I decide that I must have been carrying them around for several miles. They must have latched on when I stopped at Pee Lane. I know the bugs were buzzing around as I stood there and I had to swat them away, but I must have missed those two. It kinda makes me laugh. I mean, I hate getting bit by those things, but it is kinda comical to think those two were holding on for dear life (kinda a pun, since they be deer flies?) as I ran, because I'm so freaking fast. But this reminds me of a few times when I take my ballcap off to swat away flies buzzing around my head, and one time, it was horse flies. These are the bigger, badder, meaner cousins of deer flies. I swatted them away with my cap, and put the cap back on my head. Guess what? Another horse fly must have snuck in just as the cap went down. Now I've got this unhappy, large thing buzzing around in the cramped space next to my scalp. Mother nature 1,000, Manley zero. At mile four, I notice a sharp pain in my right wrist. What is going on with that? I know my wrists are weak from too much computer and video game use, but why would it pop up during a run? All you need to do is come along for the ride, Mr. Wrist. You don't do anything else. Just chill out, okay? I think the pain goes away after a bit. Sometimes there are cars passing within ten to twenty feet of me as I make my turn at the end of my road, and I wonder what those car people think. Do they hate me because I'm there exercising? Do they get inspired to see me running? Maybe they go home and decide to go out for a walk or jog or something active? Maybe I'm making a difference in their lives just by being myself and exercising for them to see? Fifty minutes have passed. I got exactly 5.80 miles again, just like day 2. That ties my longest distance this month, and I'm very happy. This day started out like it could be trouble, but I ended up having a good showing.

POST-RUN: I walk to my blacktop driveway for stretching. I notice I am not breathing hard for the second day in a row, so I think that helps solidify in my mind that I am making progress and my heart and lungs are getting stronger. My back doesn't decompress when I do my waist bend. No cracking or vertebrae pulling apart. But I can feel that they should do that, but it just won't give. I do get some knee cracks when I bend down and stretch into some yoga dog things. The blacktop feels cool. That is great. I've had it so hot sometimes that it hurt to be in contact for more than a few seconds. No bugs are near me while I laid down to stretch out my quads. Maybe those two deer flies told their friends that enough was enough today. Either way, I'm grateful. I get up and walk to my house. I close my eyes for a bit and almost run into the rain barrel by my garage. Easy there, little fella. Don't kill yourself after the run. Wait for tomorrow's run. As I head inside, I look at my forearms and notice two or three little black flies are caught in my wet arm hair. They are trapped in the sweaty hair forest. If I could zoom in on their faces, would there be looks of pure happiness or pure horror? Either way, Mother Nature 1,001, Manley zero. My weight after a shower was 166.8 pounds (up 0.2).

Wednesday, July 5 from 6:29 AM to 7:19 AM

Splits	Time	Cumulative Time	Distance
1	8:14.0	08:14	1.00
2	8:21.9	16:36	1.00
3	8:20.5	24:56	1.00
4	8:32.1	33:28	1.00
5	8:29.2	41:58	1.00
6	8:02.8	50:00	0.99
Summary	50:00	50:00	5.99 mi
Average Pace 8:21 min/mi			

PRE-RUN: I wore my green ninja turtle pants, blue t-shirt, white socks, Garmin watch, ballcap, and decided to wear my black hood. I checked the sky outside before leaving the house and saw the wind just blowing hard, and the clouds covering the sky. I decide to not put on any sunscreen, and my armpits didn't hurt or sting, so I didn't do any petroleum jelly. I think it was my old deodorant, so I've changed that for good now. I see a bunch of crows out on my driveway talking and gabbing with each other. They look like they're having fun. They must have had their coffee already. I figured it would be cold outside, so I grabbed my black hood. Last night, I didn't do myself any favors. I pigged out for the 4th of July. Two huge cheeseburgers and fries, 20 cookies, a big bowl of ice cream, candy, and probably 8 cups of milk. During morning stretches, my left Achilles tendon caught for a bit. Almost like there is a knot in there, and then as I stretch it out, the knot catches and finally goes over a hump or untangles. But I can reproduce it over and over, so that is weird. It doesn't hurt, but feels strange and like my body shouldn't be able to do that. It wouldn't be the only thing weird about my body, let me tell you. But I won't tell you, because I have a limit to my shame. Even before I'm out the door, I have "Hungry Eyes" in my head. *I look at you and I fantasize. I got, hungry eyes.* Oh, and those saxophones in that melody bounce around in my head as I go to my driveway for some final psyching up and deep breathing. But, I have to work today, so I need to get going. I can't dawdle.

RUNNING: I start out and the first mile pretty much flies by. I think my body is on auto-pilot. Sometimes I do that just to see what happens and feel what my body thinks is good. Like my body can do its thing, and that allows my mind to be free-flowing and think about whatever. I don't even look at my watch once. I don't want to see my time or pace or anything yet. Sometimes it takes a lot of mental energy to not look at your watch. It is so tempting, but I persevere. I hear the beep of one mile done. Now, I look at my watch at that moment and see an 8:14 split. Woah, that is surprising. I didn't think I was going that fast. And is that good or bad? Will I be able to make it through the rest of the 42 minutes? Was I unconsciously going faster for...what exactly? Or maybe this is just normal for today. I kinda think that is weird because of all the extra food crap I ate yesterday. But maybe yesterday's food won't affect me until tomorrow. That'll be interesting to see what happens tomorrow. As I finish that first mile, I notice two flies are following me. They look big and black. Probably my deer fly buddies from past days. My very own wingmen, I guess. They get close to trying to land on me, but basically just fly circles around me as I run circles around the loop. Kinda funny to wonder what the flies are thinking? I mean, their life is already so short, and they are spending hours of it with me? I'm flattered. Also, if their lives are so short and they reproduce quickly, I guess it is technically possible that on July 1st, I was running with Mr. Frank Fly, and then by July 31st, I will be running with Frank's great-great-granddaughter Cher Fly. I don't see any animals besides the occasional bird. Those crows from earlier are long gone. I don't see any fresh animal landmines either. I wonder if all the fireworks noise from last night scattered the animals? We didn't do any fireworks ourselves, but the neighbors did plenty for the entire neighborhood. Tom Petty stops by in my head. *Yeah running down a dream, that never would come to me and working on a mystery, running down a dream.* Pretty appropriate today. Because of the running, in case you didn't get it. The second mile beeps and I look down at my watch. It is 8:21. Very nice, two good miles in a row and I'm not really forcing anything. Today might be a new high-mileage day. It was just 5.80 the other day, and I think I'm ahead of that. The sun never did come out. The clouds kept moving and the whole landscape was gray and dim. Well, I guess I can't pretend to be Superman today. No yellow sun to suck energy from. Nonetheless, my black hood soon feels like a wet towel stuck to my head. But with mile 3 done and a split time of 8:20, I don't feel like taking it off and messing up any karma or whatever might be in play. At about 3.3 miles, my left hip introduces itself to me with a good stabbing pain right in front. I gingerly touch it with my left hand and can feel the huge hip tendon or whatever moving as my leg runs. It must be getting tweaked or worn out. The pain isn't awful, so I press on and it goes away after a few more laps. I try out some butt kicks and high knees. I can feel the left hip hurt and pull during the middle of the high knees, but the pain goes away after another bunch of steps and I forget about it for the time being. At mile 4 my bug brothers are back. Flying around and doing aerial acrobatics. Are they showing off for me, or just lulling me into a false sense of security so they can attack? Almost as if on cue, I feel something on my back. A quick swat, but I'm not sure what it was. At my normal turn around spot by the highway, there is a gray truck stopped at the stop sign and I wave to him. It takes the male driver an extra second or two, but he does wave back. Maybe he doesn't get waves very often? Maybe he didn't understand what I was for a bit? I wonder if I might be the only stranger that smiles and waves to him today. Does that make him happier today?

Did I have any impact on his life, or am I forgotten as soon as he turns onto the highway and turns his attention to the rest of the day? During mile 5, I feel a heavy bug on my left ear. I'm still wearing my ball cap over my black hood, so the bug is actually on the hood fabric. For a split second, it feels like it is doing spins in a circle, or maybe gymnastics. I instantly think about Princess Leia's head buns. And then it flits away without a swat from me. Maybe my wingmen told it to get lost? And then I feel what I hope is a large bead of sweat fall into my left ear canal. My gosh, it better just be sweat. My hood is still on, so no way something else got into my ear, right? But maybe that bug jostled my hood fabric enough to get a drop of sweat to move into my ear. Thanks bug. I look at my watch. I'm at 5.5 miles and have about 4 minutes left. I think this is going to be my highest mileage day this month. I might even get close to 6 miles. I can barely feel I am going faster. I still don't need to expend lots of mental energy, but I can tell I'm into this run now. I like the idea of getting further today than 5.8, so I kinda kick it in a bit. Whenever I consciously make my legs faster, I have to pump my arms harder. Those are the body blows I'm throwing against the earth or air or whatever. My invisible opponent. And as my legs go faster, I feel like a cartoon animal that start to run fast and their legs turn into circle blurs. Like Bugs Bunny or Wile E Coyote or whatever. I feel like a cartoon and think my legs are way out in front of my body. I must look ridiculous. I look at my legs as they turn over, again not super-fast, but faster than earlier. Watching your own legs run from above is almost alien. They appear and disappear over and over. My feet don't look right. They can't possibly be touching down on the road correctly. But they do, just in time, they do and I don't fall. Balance is pretty amazing. *Running down a dream, something something mystery, running down a dream.* Oh Manley, don't watch your legs, keep your eyes on the road. My body is drifting to the edge of the road. I head back to the middle again. I started running in the middle yesterday and kept at it today. I think I'll keep in the middle for the rest of the runs; it seems like it is saving me some wear and tear on my body on this township gravel road. Watch the watch. Fifty minutes almost up. Finger on the button. 49:58, 49:59, 50:00. Stop the clock. Oh, my gosh, I can't believe it. The mileage is stuck at 5.99 miles. Unbelievable, I couldn't get another .01 miles anywhere in 50 minutes. I've never had that happen before, so comically short of something. I look at my watch and notice mile 4 was the longest. What, I couldn't go a little faster there to get the extra .01? Oh well, don't dwell on negatives. This is really a positive. You just blew up your long distance this month. You jumped up from 5.80 to 5.99 in the same time frame. Now, keep at it and improve again and again.

POST-RUN: Not breathing hard, but I do take some nice slow, deep breaths to try to get back to normal breathing. I walk to my blacktop driveway and smirk. There on the driveway is my body's sweat stain from yesterday's run. I think what the heck and stand in the same spot for my stretches. Might as well give the blacktop a double dose of Manleyness. My back stretch goes well. I feel two vertebrae pull out and feel that void again. It is like a locked-up pressure getting released. It feels good. I pull off my ball cap and black hood and feel the cool air on my sweaty head. That feels good. I have sweat in my eyes from being on the ground, so I wipe my entire face and forehead with my t-shirt. And wouldn't you know it, as I wipe my forehead, I feel a heavy thing on the fabric, and it rolls over and over as the fabric is moved across my head. I look down at my shirt, and there is a stupid deer fly struggling to fly away. In that little second from taking my cap and hood off to wiping my face, a deer fly went in for the kill. What, is my disgusting sweat a sweet elixir that they all crave? Am I their fountain of youth? I flick the wounded fly away with my finger and walk into the house. I figure that last deer fly was Mother Nature getting one more shot in on me before I leave. Okay, okay, I'm going. I've overstayed my welcome. I get it. My weight after a shower was 165.4 pounds (down 1.4).

Thursday, July 6 from 6:54 AM to 7:44 AM

Splits	Time	Cumulative Time	Distance
1	8:14.7	08:14	1.00
2	8:13.3	16:28	1.00
3	8:17.3	24:45	1.00
4	8:21.5	33:07	1.00
5	8:18.4	41:26	1.00
6	8:04.7	49:31	1.00
7	0:30.0	50:01	0.06
Summary	50:01	50:01	6.06 mi
Average Pace 8:15 min/mi			

PRE-RUN: Woke up around 5:45 AM today. It was dark outside. Lots of cloud cover and rain looked imminent. My weather app said only 10% chance of rain this morning for the next few hours, so I decided to run. I didn't need any sunscreen and decided on no hood today. I wore blue Batman pajama pants and a blue t-shirt and ball cap. I was still excited about my run yesterday, but I felt stiff. I took my time and did my morning stretches and had my one cup of coffee.

RUNNING: I walked outside and it seemed even darker that before. It was like someone shut the world's lights off. Or put them on dim. Peter Droge's song popped into my head. *If you don't love me, I'll kill myself. If you don't love me, I'll kill myself.* Obviously, a moody song. Kinda appropriate for the dark, moody running atmosphere today, though.

Body status check: Nothing feels bad, nothing feels wrong. Good start. First mile is going well. I have decided not to look at my pace or time at all, just to see what my body does. Going down the curve on the west side of the loop, there are two bunnies, about fifty feet apart. Both let me get close, maybe only 5 to 10 feet away, before they hop into the underbrush and weeds on side of the road. I get my first deer fly bite on my left shoulder. One swat and it falls to the gravel as I keep running. The first mile beeps and it is 8:14. Not bad, not bad, that is just like yesterday, give or take a second. One mile done. And then I feel a drop, two drops, a light mist. My 10% chance of rain has now become 100%. Of course, just my luck. But it isn't too bad. But the humidity is high, I can easily tell because I've wiped off my face at least three times during the first mile, and usually I don't wipe the first time until well into the second mile. I can see the sky, mostly all clouds, but now there is a blade of sun, a horizontal sliver of sun parked right between two large mountains of clouds. It looks like a sun sandwich. As big and powerful as the sun is, I don't think it will win this battle. All these clouds look too big and too thick. I've resigned myself to running in dim light for the next 40 minutes. At about the 1.5 miles mark, I see a nasty looking jagged horizontal streak of lightning. I listen for the thunder, but hear nothing. Maybe it is that heat lightning I've heard about. If there is thunder, I'm going to have to call this off. As much as I would hate stopping, I don't want to be struck by lightning. But I still hear no thunder. And I only saw that one bolt. It looked like that zig zag on Charlie Brown's t-shirt. The mist is steady but not heavy. It is actually kinda fun and refreshing. And when I do my big turnaround at the highway spot, there are no cars or trucks. No sounds, just a slight wind and the mist, and I take a deep breath. It is wonderful. So new and fresh and beautiful and wonderful, I wish I could put it in a bottle. And then it is gone as my shoes hit the gravel and I run up the road back to my loop. At this point, about 2 miles in, I notice my Batman pajama pants are heavy. They are laden with sweat and rain, I guess. The humidity is high. It isn't awful because the temperature isn't high, but the humidity is definitely making itself known. I feel like I am carrying a couple of water jugs on my legs. Maybe some saddlebags. Mile 2 beeps and it is another good time, 8:13. Hmm, not bad. Another lightning bolt flashes in the sky. Oh, I suppose this will start out to be a great run, and I'll have to quit. That seems about right. But no thunder again. That gives me hope. So, I dig down and keep running. There are no animals out, except a few birds that fly in front of me once in a while. No neighbor dogs barking. I hear one neighbor's outside A/C unit rattling as I run by her house. The light gray gravel is turning darker in spots as the watery mist accumulates here and there. Almost done with mile two and my lower right belly aches. Feels like a pressure, something in there. I figure it is my body getting revenge for all the crap I put in it.

Just last night I ate like 14 pizza rolls, a big cup of ice cream, two big turkey sandwiches, and milk and pop. Oh, and several cookies. I don't know why I continue to do this. My belly ache shifts a bit, but hangs on tight to the lower right side. Screw you, it says. I think I better make some signs and tape them to the snack food cupboard or something. Maybe a subtle, "Hey fatso" or "Yo, dolt, quit eating this junk." Maybe it would stop me, maybe, but I'm not sure. My legs feel good. Nothing else stands out as an issue. I consciously splay out my fingers on both hands, as then it helps me splay out my toes in my shoes. I want to make sure I'm getting a good flat strike on the road. I want to hit the road with part of my midfoot and part of my forefoot, and I think this helps. Another half a mile and my belly ache now sits in the low middle. It feels like I'm wearing a fanny pack. Now, I've got two fannies, one in front and one in back. I feel bloated. And then I am saved. I know I'm the only one outside right now, but I hear the sweet, sweet notes of a trumpet behind me. I look behind me, but there's nothing there. And suddenly my belly ache is almost gone. Running is not glamorous. It just is. Mile three beeps and another good time is posted. I decide to not let up. Whatever speed I'm going at, just keep it up. Don't look at my watch anymore, but you got a chance to beat your distance from yesterday. Your hilarious 5.99 miles. During mile 4, the gravel is mostly dry again. How is that possible? Am I sucking up the rain as I run over it? That might be it, because my shirt is completely soaked. The sweat stain in front that usually sits on my sternum is across the entire shirt. I cannot use it to wipe my face much anymore. And I know my back is soaked. It feels like I'm carrying a water balloon back there. I pull my shirt away from my back skin, and wouldn't you know it. There's a deer fly on my right shoulder this time, just sucking my life away. How long has he been there? Jeez Louise. Now, I find myself checking my face and neck and shoulders more often. The wind picks up again, and I swear I run into a head wind the entire way around the loop. How is that even possible? I feel like Kramer lost in downtown New York: He calls Jerry and says how can first street and first street intersect itself? I must be at the nexus of the universe. Maybe my loop is the nexus today. A wind from all 360 degrees of a circle. I meet a truck with headlights at my highway turnaround. I cannot see inside, the lights are too bright, but I smile and wave as I turn around. I have no idea if they saw me. Can't worry about it, just keep running. Take some deep breaths, slow your breathing down, gather your energy. One mental trick that I made up is to breathe out of my mouth slightly slower than normal breathing and pretend I am shooting Link's hook shot (from Legend of Zelda games) out into the road about 10 or 20 feet ahead. Then I close my mouth and breathe in deep with my nose, imagining that the rope from the hook shot is being reeled back into my head, pulling me forward at a faster speed. So, subconsciously, I run a little faster as that rope is pulled back in, and I calm down my breathing a bit. I smell a wonderful fragrance just for a second. It was either flowers or trees or berries, I don't know what. Just bountiful and tasty and aromatic, but then gone. No idea where that came from. I suppose I could have hallucinated it? *And if you don't love me, I'll kill myself.* I see a big mommy turkey and two little ones out on the highway, scooting across to my side. I clap my hands, try to spook them to go faster. There are cars coming on the highway, but the turkeys make it in time. Time has flown by, miles have flown by, I check my watch, I can't miss the 50-minute stoppage. I see I have a little over a minute left and I'm at 5.95 miles. I know I can beat yesterday's distance now. Just keep on running. In fact, run a little faster. Leave nothing to chance. Fifty minutes and I'm done. 6.06 miles. All right, that's great. That beats my 5.99 from yesterday. My new top distance. But wow, even that was just an 8:15 average pace, and not close enough to my 7:47 pace needed for my 10K record. Well, who cares, you weren't going for the 10K record today, so chill out. Walk home.

POST-RUN: I walk onto my blacktop driveway. The rain has now just started to pick up. The drops are bigger. That is awesome that it waited until I was done. Now, I do my stretches. My back is tight, and the stretch feels great. I can still see my sweat stain on the blacktop from yesterday, but with this rain, that'll be gone soon. I take a few steps to the left and decide to make a new sweat angel. I lay on my belly to stretch my quads and hips. There is no sun, only clouds, and the rain is beating on my face. I feel great. I close my eyes and just feel the world, feel nature. I might be the only one in the entire world right now stretching their legs in the rain. I push myself up and stand up. I look at my watch history and see that mile 4 was the slowest mile. Wasn't that the case yesterday, too? Hmm, maybe I should pay attention to that tomorrow. When mile 4 starts, maybe I'll switch my watch to mile pace and make sure that I keep it up. I wonder why mile 4 is the slowest. That is intriguing, because mile 5 and mile 6 were good and great, respectively. Body status check: All seems good, no obvious leg issues. Arm pits feel fine. Belly ache is long gone. My weight after a shower was 166.2 pounds (up 0.8).

Friday, July 7 from 6:32 AM to 7:22 AM

Splits	Time	Cumulative Time	Distance
1	8:05.4	08:05	1.00
2	7:47.3	15:53	1.00
3	7:55.7	23:48	1.00
4	7:46.9	31:35	1.00
5	7:48.1	39:23	1.00
6	7:35.1	46:59	1.00
7	3:03.0	50:01	0.42
Summary	50:01	50:01	6.42 mi
Average Pace 7:48 min/mi			

PRE-RUN: There was a big storm last night, lots of rain and thunder and lightning. Ground looks wet. Sun is starting to peek out. Not very many clouds. Should be a sunny run. Haven't even started running yet and I've got *Give me some good news baby, the world's gone crazy, give me some good news baby, give it to me, give it to me* stuck in my head. I am wearing my blue t-shirt, blue shorts, white socks, Garmin watch, baseball cap, and no hood. I put sunscreen all over my face and neck and legs and arms. I look in the mirror and it looks like I'm dressing up like a clown. Pure white base makeup. But, I'd rather do this than get skin cancer. I drank one cup of coffee and started to stretch inside a bit, then went outside to stretch in the driveway. It was a good temperature, little bit of wind, and looking to be a beautiful day. But suddenly I didn't want to run. I was walking around in circles in my driveway, I guess breathing deeply, trying to get ready, but I didn't want to go. I think I did so well yesterday with a new top distance that I didn't want to try that hard again. I didn't want to get less than that and feel like a failure. Also, there is a constant growling sound that I didn't notice right away, but now it is impossible to ignore. It takes me a few seconds, but then I see the smoke curling in the sky away in the distance. The county's blacktop mixing plant must be operating. It is about a mile away, as the crow flies, but it rumbles and rumbles. Like some distant thunder that never stops. But finally, I just didn't think anymore and pressed the button on my watch and started running.

RUNNING: I noticed three bunnies right away. Two were in my front yard and one was on the loop on the edge of the gravel. If there are three bunnies now, I shudder to think how many bunnies there will be at the end of this month. I might have to run on their backs if they keep multiplying. The bunny on the road immediately runs away and jumps in the bushes as I get close. Body status check: No pain, things feel pretty good, maybe just a small lingering of weariness from yesterday's hard run. Otherwise, I feel good and keep on trucking. The sun is definitely out. Nothing but blue skies now. No clouds. I breathe deep as I run, shoot out a few hook shots from my mouth for fun to keep in the game. I see a turkey on the western curve of the loop. He casually walks into the neighbor's yard and hides behind a tree. He watches as I go by to make sure I'm not much of a threat. It's a big turkey with a beard, and he's probably up to my waist. I'm just glad he didn't chase after me. I've never had that happen and don't want to start now. I have no idea what I would do if one chased after me. They are fast, and I don't think I could outrun him. Luckily, he seems more afraid of me. There are lots of animal tracks in the soft dirt of the loop. The rain has mostly dried up, but the dirt road is just slightly spongy. And the animals must have been on the move after the storm broke last night. I see tons of deer and turkey prints, and there is even some kind of small bear or big dog or something with a paw print. Just a single print, didn't notice any others. Part of the curve on the western side is illuminated by the sun as I run up to it. There are hundreds of little green plants (probably baby weeds) growing up all over that part of the road. With the rain or dew all over them and the sun shining, they look like hundreds of light green emeralds waiting to be picked up. It's really pretty. I run over the top of them, imagining I'm running on a green carpet. At my highway turnaround spot, I suck in a deep breath with my nose, and it is putrid. The strong smell of oil and rubber and blacktop and whatever fills my face. Yuck, that stupid blacktop mixing plant. It seems like something always ruins a perfect running day. Thankfully, the smell is somehow only saturated around that turnaround. It doesn't smell like that on the loop anywhere. So, onward I go. My first mile beeps and I look at my watch for the first time. Hmm, an 8:05. That's unexpected. I didn't think I was going that fast, but I'll take it. I wipe my face with my shirt. The humidity isn't too bad, but I can tell my shirt will be soaked at the end, like normal. Now I'm running counterclockwise around the northwest curve and that same turkey is in the road again. He must have decided he was too cool to hide behind the neighbor's tree again. He takes off on a trot and before I know it, I'm chasing him down the road. A full-grown man running, basically following a full grown turkey down a dirt road. Who's the real turkey? The tom puts on a burst of speed and turns down Pee Lane. That's where we part ways, I guess. It is pretty cool to see turkeys run. I can imagine them as little dinosaurs. It is similar to how the velociraptors run in Jurassic Park movies. And amazingly, no bugs yet. I haven't seen one fly by, none have landed on me, I don't hear them in the weeds. Maybe the storm blew them away? Mile 2 beeps and huge shocker, it reads 7:47. That is way faster than I realized. I wasn't consciously trying for that, but I wasn't relaxing either. Big surprise. Two miles down, 4 to go, and I wonder what I've started here. Should I try for the same speed and time for this third mile? I guess so. Why not? At my current pace, I'm even ahead of yesterday's awesome run. I must feel good or something. I am wearing shorts and no black hood. The wind is cool on my sweaty skin. I think I'm

46

going to try for something here, I don't know what, though. We'll see how mile 3 turns out. I'm concentrating now. I'm not just running on auto-pilot. I think my body is tired from the last 2 miles and I concentrate to keep the pace. Breathe out, hook shot, breathe in, wind that rope back in. Hook shot, hook shot. My mind is in the game now, and that's not a great place to be. When you have to concentrate on each step, each breath, each movement and foot strike and stride, then the run seems longer. But, I did this to myself. This third mile takes a while. I'm breathing hard and sweating. Multiple face swipes with my shirt. Mile 3 beeps and boom, a 7:55 mile. Slower than the last one, but still good. Now, I'm trying to think what my previous 10K PR pace was. My mind draws a blank. I know it was under-8-minute miles, but I can't remember. Was it 7:55 or 7:51 or 7:41? Oh geez, why can't I remember? You'd think I'd have that tattooed across my brain, since this whole July running goal of running every single day morphed into having a secondary goal of beating my previous 10K time. You would think that I would know the freaking pace to beat, but my mind is blank. I am trying so hard to run fast. And now I'm into mile 4 and I remember yesterday's thoughts. Mile 4 for the last two days has been my slowest. I must have eased off the gas or something, but I don't want that to happen today. I've got three great mile times in, half way done to a 10K, let's go get it. Give mile 4 my best, don't let it be my worst, and I'll go from there.

If I have a good time, then I'm going for it. If not, then I'll ease down and not kill myself. It all hinges on mile 4 now. And my fragile brain, because I'm still running fast and it hurts. My left hip starts to nag at me. Then, my left knee nags at me. I don't even think about doing butt kicks or high knees. I can barely think about anything other than breathe in, breathe out, step, push, step, push. I'm not happy right now. This kinda sucks. My chest is hurting from all the deep breathing and constant hard breathing. Hook shot, hook shot, hook shot. *I got some bad news baby, give me some good news baby.* The song is fleeting, it can't grab any traction. My mind cannot afford the brain cells to even get the lyrics right. I pump my arms to get my legs going when I notice they might be lagging. Body blow, body blow, throw a haymaker. Keep these stupid legs going, come on, come on. I've turned my watch to show my current mile pace. I need to know, I need to watch it. It seems like every 10 steps I glance down at my watch to see my pace. I've made myself into a monster. I don't like running anymore. This sucks, and I want to stop. Why'd I do this to myself? Oh, just shut up, shut up, keep running. Why stop now? Only a few miles left, forget about it, look over there, I'm passing Pee Lane again for the umpteenth time and I see the big turkey sitting down in the middle of the road. I've never ever seen that before, come to think of it. I've never seen a turkey sit. They've always been walking or running or even flying short distances. What is that turkey doing? It is so comical. Big fat body, tiny head and neck looking around. He probably thinks I look stupid too. I feel stupid. My breathing is hard, and I work to calm myself down over and over. Breathe slower. Then, slower, again, slower. Keep going. Keep pumping your arms. I know this is uncomfortable. Okay, mile 4 is about to beep. Oh, yes, a 7:47. Yes, this is it, this is it. I blew the last two days' mile 4 out of the water. I am well under 8 minute miles. I think my previous 10K was 7:47 minute miles. Go for it, go for it, I will have to run faster. Get going. Mile 5 is underway and I cannot give up now. No way. Keep going. Hook shot, hook shot, hook shot. Gosh darn it, this hurts. I hate this. My right foot hurts now. Do your splay technique to fix your strike zone. I splay out both my hands to force my toes to splay out. For a few foot strikes, I can feel my right forefoot is hitting the ground flush. It is an improvement, but I can't think about that anymore. Keep breathing or I am going to die. I don't even pay attention to my surroundings anymore. It is just me, my watch, and the loop. The gosh darn stupid loop. I make my turnaround at the highway and get a face full of that blacktop crap smell again. It is awful, and not what I need in my face right now. Look at my watch, see my pace, still hovering around the 7:45 area, that's great. But this still sucks, it is hard, and I want to stop. No, I am not freaking stopping. Just imagine the end. Imagine getting the PR record. I can tell my wife, my kids, I can put it on my blog. Just keep running.

Hook shot, splay your toes, pump your arms, wipe your face, hook shot, breathe, breathe, just freaking keep breathing and moving. I'm concentrating so hard on my body to keep going, that I don't even register the beep on my watch. By the time I realize my watch made a noise, I look down and see I'm at 6.03 miles and the time is around 47 minutes. Holy crap, I am going to do it. I've got less than three minutes but I'm already over 6 miles and almost to 10K distance. Do. Not. Stop. Please keep going. This is so painful, but do not stop. Keep breathing, you stupid jerk, breathe in and out. My legs start going slightly faster, I want this now. I still hate it and want to stop, but I don't. I want this 10K PR record today. I'm not going to waste this opportunity, not a chance. My head whips back and forth between the loop and the watch. At 6.20 miles, my watch reads 48:19 and my mind screams YES. Yes, you magnificent idiot, you did it. You got it, you got it, you got it. Wait, why are you still running. You can stop now. Oh, shoot, no I can't. I'm supposed to go to 50 minutes every day. Gosh dang it. This sucks. I want to stop. This last two minutes is taking forever, but around the loop I go. I can't stop now. I see 6.30 go by, then 6.35 miles, and still I have time left. Why? Will you please be done, for the love of Pete? I want to quit running right now. This is awful. My lungs and chest are done. My legs are done. I start to feel those pins and needles in my lower legs. I get those at points like this. Too much for me. Please stop. I start to slow down and almost start walking when the watch still shows 49:56, 49:57. Please be done. One more huge breath. Fifty minutes. I went 6.42 miles. That is so huge, so awesome, way over what I thought I could do. It is over, thank you, thank you, thank you, it is over. You did it. You did it. I'm on the part of the loop that is farthest from my house. I walk and walk. Catch my breath. This is my freaking victory lap.

POST-RUN: It takes many minutes for me to get to my driveway for stretching. I take my ball cap off. It feels like it weighs ten pounds from all the sweat. My blue shirt is dark with sweat. I notice I have little black specks and flecks in my leg hair. All the dirt and dust and little pebbles probably flew up off the road and clung for the whole run. I absolutely did not start out today thinking I could break my 10K PR. In fact, I was hemming and hawing before even running. I didn't want to even start. I was afraid. Afraid of it being too hard. Fifty minutes is a long time. If I don't think about it, then I can do it. But if I start thinking about how long 50 minutes really is, then I'm in trouble. Wow, this run really shows how important pace is. My first mile was the slowest, but it got me started. If that 8:05 would have been an 8:35, I never would have given my 10K record a thought. But then my mile 2 and 3 paces were great, and I just knew. I had to try. I'm glad I did. It was awful. It was hard. But I got it. I got my record. And just to make sure I didn't forget about Mother Nature, I swear to God a stupid deer fly landed on my front left shoulder while I was stretching my legs. I didn't see it or feel it in time. It bit me, so I nailed it. The deer flies don't stop around here, I guess. So, why should I? My weight after a shower was 165.2 pounds (down 1.0).

Saturday, July 8 from 8:18 AM to 9:08 AM

Splits	Time	Cumulative Time	Distance
1	8:12.1	08:12	1.00
2	8:10.3	16:22	1.00
3	8:19.7	24:42	1.00
4	8:19.3	33:01	1.00
5	8:29.0	41:30	1.00
6	8:18.2	49:49	1.00
7	0:11.8	50:00	0.02
Summary	50:00	50:00	6.02 mi
Average Pace 8:18 min/mi			

PRE-RUN: After the high of a successful run and PR wore off yesterday, my body kinda gave me a wake-up call in the middle day and said don't forget about me. I experienced charley horses in my left quad, my right hamstring, and in between the toes of my right foot. Thankfully, they didn't all occur at once or I might have shriveled up into a woebegone meat sack. The right hamstring attack happened while sitting down at work, and the quad and toes happened later that night at home. I stretched them out the best I could, but everything felt sore and worn out. I woke up today later than normal as it is the weekend. I was up around 7 AM and had a single cup of coffee. I checked my legs, and they weren't too bad, little sore. My lower back felt bad though. I did my morning stretches. I wore my green ninja turtle pants, dark blue shirt, and ball cap. The sun is out in full force and there are no clouds in the sky. I lather up in my sunscreen/clown pancake makeup. I keep thinking about what I should run today. There is no way I'm going to try for a PR or anything today. I need a recovery day, especially with my legs and back feeling gingerly. I decide that I should still try to get to 6 miles every day. That is about an 8:20 per mile pace. I think 6 miles is a good goal, but it is pretty stupid that only 8 days into my goal (out of 31 days in July) I keep changing things around. If you remember, I started out at 9 minute per mile pace as my goal, now I'm shooting for 40 seconds under that every mile. Not sure if I'm making the right choice; obviously I'm in this for the long haul. I still have 23 more days after today. I cannot prematurely kill myself and leave nothing left in my body to tackle the half-marathon on the 31st. But in the end, I decide to go for the 6 miles.

RUNNING: The first thing I notice is no blacktop mixing plant smell and no loud rumbling noise. It is Saturday and the county workers are off duty. The little wins are important. On the downside, I immediately notice there is a lot more people-activity outside than usual. Probably because of the weekend and my later start. My southern neighbor is driving around the loop in his giant blue tractor heading to a back field to play farmer. He's from a big city down south, and he has a cabin up here by our house. His cabin is bigger than our house. I look to the highway and lots of cars and trucks are moving. Lots are pulling campers and boats, trying to get someplace for the day. I finish a few more calf stretches and press go on my watch. I start out slowly trying to get my body moving. Boy, the sun is bright. No clouds, just pure blue sky. The gravel is bright and gray-white, the sun reflects off it pretty well. I press the button on my watch to make sure my current mile pace is visible. I decide I'm going to have to keep a close eye on that during this run. Six miles to go, that's it. Ha-ha, good luck. I can already feel my left calf muscle screaming at me. With every step on the gravel it pulls and tweaks and bothers me. A good muscle is a quiet muscle. Just keeps its head down and does its work and never complains. This left calf muscle is complaining. Hey, buddy, guess what, it says. I hate you. I hate you. I hate you. I'm only half way around one loop lap and my left quad jumps into the game. Two problems in one leg. Not a good sign. I concentrate to keep my stride normal. I splay out my fingers to splay out my toes. I want to help myself the best I can. Do good foot strikes. Keep up a consistent stride. Keep to the middle of the road. Pump your arms. Yeah, but how about I just jump off your femur and fall on the road, my left quad says. Every step feels like my quad wants to do just that. I imagine it bursting out of my skin and landing on the gravel and running ahead, leaving me to chase after it with one leg. Why, quad, why do this to me? Just do your job. On the gravel, up ahead on the southwestern curve of the loop, I see a dark greenish, blackish something in the dirt. I run by it and it looks like a dead toad. And not fresh either. Just a quick glance, but looks lumpy and soupy and friendless. But now I wonder if it wasn't a dead toad. Maybe it was a poop pile. Boy, I'll have to pay attention next lap. Until then, I won't know. Mile 1 beeps. I've been watching my pace, and 8:12 flashes across the screen. Good, good start. I mean, my legs are bad, but I just built myself an 8 second lead, if I'm shooting for 8:20 per mile. Lots of birds outside, flying around. The air is fresh and cool. I suck in a deep breath and the coolness is exciting. Robins fly into and out of the tall grass along the loop. I don't see a turkey, though, and then I do. As I run past Pee Lane, way at the far end, a large fat turkey is standing there looking over the field. It looks like a sentry. Is it the same turkey from yesterday? I don't know. But it looks majestic in a turkey sort of way. At my highway turnaround, I have to cut it short and quick as there are too many cars bearing down on the intersection. I don't want to get hit by the vehicles or rocks that get kicked up or give the drivers something to worry about. I hear the low rumble of the neighbor's blue tractor coming back out of his field and heading around the loop. He's going on the same side I have to run on next, so we are on a collision course. He isn't looking my way, so for a split second I wonder if he ran me over, would he even know. The freaking tires are taller than I am. I think the whole thing is 8 feet tall. I start friendly waving, he sees me and gives me a big slow wave back. He's got tall black and white hair like Jay Leno. Jay Leno is farming by my house. And he almost ran me over. No joke in that. Body status check: My left leg has settled down a bit, either the muscles in my calf and quad are warmed up and kinda okay, or my pain receptors said screw it and decided to stop sending impulses. But I notice the bottom of my right foot is sore or something. Not necessarily hurt, but I can feel it. And I don't want to feel it. It should just do its job. I went to a local foot doctor about three years ago, because I was new to running. I figured I was wearing the wrong shoes and doing everything else wrong. I had pains in both feet and knees. He took x-rays of my feet and watched me walk and jump and move. He looked at me and said these are the worst feet in the world for running. Turns out he was a veterinarian. Just joking, but I'll be here all night folks. He really did say I had bad feet though. If you keep running, you will regret it. You will have pain the rest of your life. I was mad. I was sad. I didn't want to stop running. And you, Mr. Doctor, can't make me. So, I did some running shoe research and decided to get neutral shoes with extra shock absorption, since at that time, I was a heavy heel striker. I still think about that doctor and what he said. I am running to be defiant to that doctor. He said stop. I didn't listen very well, did I? I run past that poop toad thing again. This time, it looks like a degraded toad. I think that long thing was a leg. Maybe, but I'm not sure. I'll check it again on the next lap. Mile 2 dings and 8:10 shows up. Now I have a good cushion, but at what expense? My left leg calf muscle acts up every so often and now my right hamstring is starting to perk up and say, don't forget about me. Jab, jab, jab. Ouch. *Turn around, every now and then I get a little bit tired of listening to the sound of my something, turn around bright eyes, total eclipse of the heart. And I need you now more than ever.* Another vehicle on the loop, this time my other neighbor is driving in a truck pulling his riding lawn mower on a trailer. Maybe he got it fixed somewhere? I wave and he waves back. I don't care for all this traffic and people stuff. For one thing, I feel like I need to wave or acknowledge all these things lest I get, oh, I don't know run over and maimed. Hook shot, keep your pace up, look at your watch, you are getting behind. Pace is 8:46 halfway through mile 3, that's not good. Get in the middle of the road, quit daydreaming, and start running. Tough it out. Get it down to 8:20. My neighbor with the truck is now on his lawn mower testing it out in his yard. I wave as I run past and he waves again. One neighbor, two vehicles, two waves. Keep running, whoa. What was that? On the western curve of the loop, a large harrier hawk swoops down right in front of me. He must have come down to about ten feet from the ground, must have spotted a meal, but then he swoops back up and in three or four giant wing flaps, he is flying away over the trees. That was cool, very beautiful bird. In and out in a few seconds, but no food for it yet. The loop is full of tractor tire marks everywhere, and they aren't great. I have to run around them, since they've marred up the gravel and I don't want to roll an ankle or something. I'm running down the road to the highway turnaround and hear a vehicle behind me coming up fast. Geez Louise, this is getting ridiculous. And who is it? My truck neighbor again, but this time he is in his red car. So, I look back and absent-mindedly wave again and he waves back. One neighbor, three different vehicles, three waves. That's enough, I think. If I see him again today, no waving. Well, maybe a head nod or something. I've wiped my face about a hundred times today. The heat is not bad, good temp, but the humidity must be really high. My shirt is soaked and still I run. I know I've lifted my shirt to expose my belly to multiple people on the highway when I do my turnarounds, so lots of people have gotten free tickets to the Manley Show. Come one, come all, step right up and see the bulbous white belly. No refunds though. Mile 4 goes by, I'm keeping my pace, but my right hamstring is still sore. My lungs feel good though. Not like yesterday's lung torture, much better today. Mile 5 is the stinging eye mile. My sweat has mixed with sunscreen and I'm partially blinded. I cannot wipe it out very well since my shirt is soaked. I try to blink and blink, eventually either I get used to the stinging or it works its way out. That didn't feel great. Next time I look at my watch, I see I'm at 5.82 miles with only a minute and a half left. That's cutting it too close, so I try to pick up the speed the best I can. My legs rebel but I just ignore it the best I can. I end at 6.02 miles for 50 minutes. Good enough for today. And I just realized no bugs at all today. That's weird.

POST-RUN: As soon as I stop running, I take a few steps while looking at my watch to see my run stats. My stomach feels yucky. I immediately think I might puke. This is a new feeling for me. I've run many times, but never felt like puking afterwards. Why now? Was it the coffee? The heat, humidity? Take some deep breaths, don't puke, don't puke. Yuck, oh, I don't feel good, but it hasn't reached DEFCON 5 mode yet. Uh, please don't barf. I walk and walk, luckily my run ended near my driveway. I stop at the end and close my eyes and just breathe. Slowly, slowly, the feeling passes. But it was close, I think, and I don't know why. Maybe dehydration? Maybe a perfect storm of body aches, humidity, sun, and whatever? I stretch my legs well, calves and quads and hamstrings. I don't want any more charley horses today. Please, please, no more. It is funny that my pace today is exactly 30 seconds slower per mile than yesterday. My forearm hair is glistening in the sun. The skin is white from sunscreen but the hairs are standing up tall. I'll have to be careful from now on. Need to stay vigilant. My body and legs are over-used, but I can't stop. I want that half-marathon PR. Stay focused. My weight after a shower was 165.0 pounds (down 0.2).

Sunday, July 9 from 6:36 AM to 7:26 AM

Splits	Time	Cumulative Time	Distance
1	8:44.7	08:44	1.00
2	8:43.2	17:28	1.00
3	8:30.1	25:58	1.00
4	8:37.7	34:36	1.00
5	8:31.5	43:07	1.00
6	6:53.7	50:01	0.83
Summary	50:01	50:01	5.83 mi
Average Pace 8:34 min/mi			

PRE-RUN: Only got about five hours of sleep last night. Ate some cookies and pizza and milk around 9:00 PM. I must have a death wish, because in hindsight, that wasn't a good move. But at the time, it made perfect sense. I woke up at 5:14 AM today, and had one cup of coffee. Did my stretches, and really tried to be slow and deliberate on my left calf muscle. It feels like a big muscle knot, and my Achilles tendon on that leg is still doing that twangy thing, where when I start to stretch it out, it feels like it unravels. Like those fake rope knots you can make, where you pull both ends and it undoes itself. I don't know what that means. It doesn't hurt, but it's a weird feeling. I wore my blue shirt, ballcap, Batman pajama pants, wasn't sure about black hood because it seemed kinda chilly outside, but the sun was shining, so I just decided on sunscreen only. It was the right choice. I'm worried about how my left calf will feel today during the run. I'm worried it

61

might pop off and lay there flopping in the dirt on the loop like some discarded fish. So, I decide to not run hard, just a normal pace and see what happens. *I want something just like this, doo-doo-doo, doo-doo-doo, where you wanna go? How much you want to risk? I want something just like this.*

RUNNING: I go outside and walk in a circle on my blacktop driveway waiting for my watch to get a GPS lock. It is sunny out with some clouds. There is a nice coolness to the air and slight wind. I psych myself up, telling me that this little run isn't going to make your calf worse, if you run smart. Watch your stride and strike and breathing. No need to win the Olympics, just finish it. *How much you want to risk? I want something just like this.* My watch finds the GPS, I press go, and I start with some careful, careful steps. It doesn't seem too bad, so I get up to normal running speed and head around the loop. I notice lots of big rocks, around golf ball-, marble-size and smaller littering the road. Then, I see the tractor marks all over. Even more than yesterday. My neighbor is ruining this road for me. Ruts and rocks, now I have to pay more attention to my foot and where it will hit the road. I don't want to sprain my ankle by stepping on a rock wrong. There are two bunnies, about twenty feet apart on the side of the road. One is obviously smaller and younger. It immediately dashes into the tall grass. The bigger, older one just kinda watches me as I run by. It follows me with one big eye and both ears.

Maybe it remembers me and isn't afraid? Maybe hoping I won't see it? I find it interesting that the bunnies have different tactics to deal with me. I look for my old friend the poop toad, but I don't see that pile of whatsit anywhere. I also notice another animal landmine is missing. I wonder where these things go. Oh, maybe my tractor neighbor ran them over and took them for a spin? Body status check: So far, so good. My left calf is still there, not screaming, but just letting me know to take it easy. My first mile comes in at 8:45. I don't like it, but I'm not gonna kill myself over it. I'm still under my 9-minute pace goal from the beginning, and this run today isn't about setting records. It is about recovery and trying to continue and be smart. I need to pick my battles and skirmishes. Know when to cut your losses and retreat. I'm not interested in everyday battles, I want to win the war. So, your 8:45 is just fine. Keep up this pace. Your calf feels better than you thought it would, right? Let it heal. I see my other neighbor's dog out in his yard. As I run by, the dog watches me, but then nonchalantly squats and tries to take a dump. He fails. I should know, since I watched him as I ran by. I think his eyes were saying, please turn away, I need some privacy, I can't go when you watch. Soon enough I'm past him and heading to the highway turnaround. There are two bugs on my shoulder, I can feel them land. Of course it would be my favorite buddies from the Deer Fly Clan. What is it with these guys? I whack them away, but one stays stuck in my shirt, so I need to pull back my finger and give it a good flick. I wonder if these deer flies are scouts for a bigger deer fly army. All good RTS players (real time strategy video game players) know you send out a few fast scouts to probe your enemies defenses and verify what they have and how much you need to bring. I wonder what the deer fly clan thinks when they keep sending out all these scouts but none return? Lots of bird sounds around the loop, but I don't actually see the birds. I turn my head to the inner circle of the loop, which is just a big prairie grass area and all the sounds stop. I find that funny. It is like those comedies where all this stuff is happening in the background, and when the main character looks over her shoulder, all the stuff stops. I keep on running. Stay in the middle of the road. Watch out for that rock. Thanks again tractor man. I should take a big shovel and dig some pot holes in his dirt driveway and see how he likes it. Or maybe dig a big pit down at the far end of Pee Lane just as it meets the farmer field and cover it with camouflage, like that little boy did in Swiss Family Robinson to catch that tiger. But in this case, I'd be catching a tractor. Maybe I'd catch him, and the next day, I would hear old Jay Leno hair softly calling out, "Hello, anybody out there. I've fallen and I can't get up." Mile two and three beep and my pace is still good. Body status check is all green. I think I feel pretty good. I mean I'm a little tired but as far as some body part screaming at me in agony, all is silent and that makes me feel relieved. The last thing I want is to have an unnecessary injury. I look at my watch and find that time has gone fast today. Only 8 minutes left, but I'm only at 4.8 miles. That's when I realize for sure I will not make 6 miles today. I mean, it was pretty easy to assume that based upon the pace, but you never really know until the math is staring you in the face. So, I just put my head down and keep breathing and running and watching my stride, stay in the middle of the loop, watch out for those rocks, keep your shoulders down. Sometimes I catch myself running with an unwanted shrug, like my shoulders are too high. So I consciously run with them forced down, not sure why they want to ride up. I wipe my face with my shirt. The sweat stain in the middle of my sternum isn't as big as it has been in the past. I guess maybe the humidity is down too. My temples by the sides of my eyes feel a little raw, it is probably a combination of sunburn, windburn, and constant face wiping. I usually put my hand underneath my shirt and start wiping from temple to temple, basically wiping my whole face in one go. Fifty minutes have passed and I'm happy with the 5.83 miles. It isn't 6, but I slow down to my walk, and I feel no pain. Nothing is more worse off than when I started, and maybe the blood pumping is helping to heal my left calf. I realize my left quad and right hamstring, so achy yesterday, didn't come up today. So that's a blessing.

POST-RUN: I get to my driveway and carefully do my hamstring and calf stretches. I bend over at the waist and watch as first one, then two, then three balls of sweat drop and splash the blacktop. I get down on all fours and arch my back first in and then out. I focus on the blacktop that is only a foot away and notice a disgusting-looking red and black spider slowing walking below my face. He is probing the space out in front of him with his two front long legs. I don't think I've seen a spider like this before, and I don't want to lie down on it when I stretch my quads. I tentatively blow some air on him to get him going. He feels it and stops and probes the ground, maybe waiting for the "wind" to die down. I don't have time for this. I blow out as hard as I can and send him flying away from my spot. I don't see where he lands or what happens, but he'll have one heck of story to tell his friends. When I stand back up from doing quad stretches, my Sweat Man outline is there in all its glory. Freshly reapplied. My Sweat Man. Is that like the Burning Man event? Could you start my sweat on fire? Probably not, but what if I was a big drinker and most of my sweat had a high alcohol content? Would it be flammable then? Well, another running day done. I am really happy with the result now. I can live with 5.83. And no extra pain, I'm liking that. I think my heart and lungs must be getting stronger after all these daily workouts. Is my little heart flexing his biceps and pumping iron as I run? Nine days done, 22 to go. *She said, where'd you want to go? How much you want to risk? I'm not looking for somebody with some superhuman gifts.* I just gotta be me. My weight after a shower was 166.8 pounds (up 1.8).

Monday, July 10 from 6:22 AM to 7:12 AM

Splits	Time	Cumulative Time	Distance
1	8:41.1	08:41	1.00
2	8:21.2	17:02	1.00
3	8:23.4	25:26	1.00
4	8:29.1	33:55	1.00
5	8:11.7	42:06	1.00
6	7:40.2	49:47	1.00
7	0:14.0	50:01	0.03
Summary	50:01	50:01	6.03 mi
Average Pace 8:18 min/mi			

PRE-RUN: I woke up at 5:34 AM and had to hurry to do my morning routine, get my 50 minute run in, and still leave on time to get to work. I wore my blue t-shirt, Batman pajama pants, and no hood. The sun was blocked by lots of clouds, so I took a chance and didn't apply any sunscreen. I felt crunched for time, so I tried to hurry and get outside. I didn't think a lot about what I wanted to accomplish. Really and truly I just wanted to get one more 50 minute run under my belt and on the books. To keep the streak alive. I had a single cup of coffee and did my body and leg stretches. Overall, I felt pretty good and nothing stood out as painful.

RUNNING: Time was short, so I did a few quick calf stretches and deep breaths. I noticed that Mother Nature left me some breakfast on my driveway. A freshly laid egg white with egg yolk bubble in the middle stared back at me. I don't know which bird left that present, but it must have been a big one. I started down the way to the highway turnaround and there were four giant black chickens standing in the road. Almost like those statue sentries in that movie *The NeverEnding Story*. I was just waiting for them to turn their eyes on me and shoot deadly lasers. But, as I ran up to them, they took off. I call them big black chickens, but they are really crows. Really big crows that, if they decided it prudent, could eat me. The clouds are keeping the sun at bay, but it looks like it might be a little dicey. It isn't complete cloud cover, and I'm beginning to think I made a big mistake by not putting sunscreen on. I don't want to stop running, but I also don't want to run in the sun for so long without protection. So far, so good, though, with the sun behind clouds, but I'll need to watch it. The clouds are organized such that some are dark black and gray and blocking all the sun light and some clouds are pure white and illuminated with the sun shining on them. It is quite the juxtaposition and really beautiful. I'm not even done with mile one and a deer fly bites me in the neck. Those are pretty painful, because the skin is so thin, and I can't see what the heck is going on back there to prevent it. I swat myself hard, which stings my neck, but at least the fly is gone. It is humid and I think the bugs have come out to play. I mean, they are really out, because I see clouds of little things floating in the air around the loop and I realize today won't be pretty. This might be a war of attrition. If I get bitten enough, there is a chance I'll go down and become a free buffet for these carnivorous monsters. I pick up the pace a bit around the curve. I don't think I want to die by bugs just yet. I glance down Pee Lane, but nothing is there on this lap. Where have the turkeys gone? Body status check: Hmm, okay, I feel good. My legs feel good, no pain. I'm glad my left calf isn't screaming out. Maybe it took a few days, but it healed up? I wonder if my left calf pain is because I'm running wrong. Maybe my stride or strike is weird. I try to pay really good attention as I run around the loop. I hold my head to the left and watch my left shoe come up off the gravel and then back down. Over and over. I think my left heel is hitting the ground too hard. I wonder if I haven't been paying very good attention the last few runs, and maybe I've been hitting the ground hard enough to damage my calf. It probably can only take so much shock and pressure. I think my left foot is hitting the heel and rolling forward to toes versus my right foot fits right in the middle with very little heel strike and rolls to the toes. Well, if that has been going on, no wonder I got injured and have nagging hip and knee issues. Time to fix this, best I can. I wish I had a coach to help with my running mechanics. I know I'm a heel striker, I figured that out about 4 years ago, which is why I've been buying and wearing Brooks Ghost shoes. I am currently running in Ghost 9. They are a neutral shoe with extra padding and sole/heel support, which I need.

The second mile beeps and I brought my pace down 20 seconds. I need to average 8:20/mile to get to 6 miles by end of 50 minutes, so I'm already behind 22 seconds from my first two miles. That's not a great start, so I better pick up the pace. *Running down a dream, never gonna see me fail, working on a mystery. Woo-hoo.* I pump my arms a little more, trying to get a kick going. I just need something to get me going. Keep your head up and straight. Stay in the middle of the road. I feel suddenly sluggish and blah. And every step I take on the loop has a little give in it, almost like I step down and then slightly slide to the side. It rained a lot yesterday, so the loop dirt must be holding the water instead of draining it. I think my body is draining water pretty good. My shirt is pretty soaked. Maybe the humidity is the silent killer? A bug bites me on the nose. Yes, the gosh dang side of my nose. I get mad and swat it away. Have these bugs no morals? Is there no part of my body off limits? I can't believe I didn't even see it in time. Maybe it snuck in when I was looking down at my shoes or something. I see some turkeys now at the end of Pee Lane. There are two full grown ones and about four little fuzzy babies. They are pretty cute. I notice some fresh deer and turkey tracks in the moist loop dirt, but I also see a few carnivore prints. I don't know what they are, but definitely bigger paw prints than cats and dogs. I hope those big turkeys keep those little babies safe. Around mile four, my wife waves to me from the living room window, and it gave me a quick burst of energy. It is our 18th wedding anniversary today, so I want to keep running as long as I can. I want to stay healthy and strong so I can make it another 18 years in this shape. Back down the loop and heading the other way, I get a feeling to pass gas. So, I start the process and then quickly stop. This feels wrong, like maybe it isn't just gas. Like maybe I should be wearing a diaper, which I'm not. I'm just running by Pee Lane, and for a split second, I think I might need to run down that track, do my business, and rechristen it as Poop Lane. But then I'm able to corral the feeling. Boy, that was a close one. I think I hit the brakes on that runaway train just in time. Maybe my cup of coffee was just too much this morning. Luckily, I won't have to rename anything today. That impromptu feeling to go has never happened to me yet, although you can imagine this has happened to plenty of other runners. Maybe they call it their brown badge of courage? I'll try to not earn that esteemed medal any time soon. As I run by my house, I hear the constant chirping of a bird. This is a relative newcomer to the area and it apparently has taken a liking to the roof of our house and our basketball hoop. A young kestrel, quite plump though, is a born killer. All worms and bugs, be afraid. But this kestrel is loud, loud, loud, and it keeps up this constant chirping, although I'm not sure who it is talking to. It is pretty cool to see it watch the grass and air and then, it quickly takes off from our roof and dive bombs to the ground and snatches its prey, usually a big juicy worm. And then flies a short distance and looks around again. Mile 5 beeps and I see I have less than 8 minutes to go a whole mile. This isn't a great situation, especially since I've been struggling all day to get near 8:20. My mile 5 pace was good at 8:11 but the previous 4 were not. That's why I'm in this hole now. But, I guess I do like challenges, especially when they are not so far out there as to be unattainable. I've run a mile in under 8 minutes before. Heck, it wasn't that long ago I got my 10K PR and I have multiple miles there that were under 8, so I know I can do it. But do I have enough in the tank for today? I pump my arms and legs faster. Two deer flies bite me in the same area of my back, which I guess is their way of cheering me on? I constantly wipe my face, trying to get going. I keep checking out my time left and distance on my watch. I am not sure I'm going to make it. Can I make it? I have to dig down deep. Come on. *I'm running down a dream, singing these words to me, trying to pick up steam, woo-hoo. I'm running down a dream.* Come on, come on, get going. Let's go. You can do this. Yes, but this really, really sucks. I'm sucking air. This last mile is torture. I am so winded. I'm not sure I'm gonna make it. It might be close. Four minutes left and just under a half mile to go. Come on, come on. Now, only 2 minutes left and a quarter mile to go. Come on, push it, push it. Breathe in and out. Pump those arms. Oh, man, finally, barely got past 6 miles before time was up. That was hard. Harder than it should have been, I think. Slow down to a walk and take it easy. The sun never came out the whole 50 minutes. Still just cloud cover. What a dreary day. But I did it once again.

POST-RUN: My breathing was heavier than usual. I completed the full 50 minutes, but it seemed like a chore. I definitely sped up on the last mile, getting a 7:40 pace, determined to get to 6 miles. It is hard for me to believe that only a few days ago I basically ran that last mile pace for the full 50 minutes. I wonder why today was so different. Sometimes it feels like I'm a different person from one day to the next. I know my body needs to recover from day to day, but I don't think I'm doing anything outlandish. I'm only 37, so I should be able to do this. I need to be able to do this. So, even though it was a slog to get to 6 miles, I did actually do it. On my driveway, I did my stretches. The bugs were bad, so of course, in my most vulnerable state where I'm face down on the blacktop and stretching my quads, two mosquitos decide to partake in their perverse blood-sucking ritual. My right shoulder takes two hits, and a third mosquito dive bombs my exposed nose and cheek. That's it, I'm done, time to head inside and get out of the war zone. My weight after a shower was 167.3 pounds (up 0.5).

Tuesday, July 11 from 6:34 AM to 7:24 AM

Splits	Time	Cumulative Time	Distance
1	9:24.3	09:24	1.00
2	9:00.2	18:25	1.00
3	8:52.3	27:17	1.00
4	8:46.2	36:03	1.00
5	8:46.2	44:49	1.00
6	5:11.6	50:01	0.65
Summary	50:01	50:01	5.65 mi
Average Pace 8:51 min/mi			

PRE-RUN: I woke up late. It was after 6 AM. I decided I had no time for coffee or much of anything else. I did some stretches and my left Achilles tendon keeps hitching. Every day now. I could just tell this whole day was going to go bad. I didn't do anything to set myself up for success. I grabbed the wrong shirt. It has a large graphic in the middle of it, right where I sweat and need to wipe my face. I hurried up and went outside, already behind schedule. I don't like the stress of knowing I need to finish this 50 minutes of exercise and then rush to a shower and work with very little time. I ran in blue shorts, ninja turtle t-shirt, and ball cap. No hood.

RUNNING: I started running. The temperature wasn't bad, and the air felt cool on my legs and arms. But the humidity was there. I ran slow. My left Achilles tendon hitched for the first 100 steps. It was distracting and worrisome. It didn't hurt exactly, but felt like it was doing the wrong thing. I wanted to run faster, but physically I just couldn't. I was probably in the 10 min/mile pace for a bit there. I looked at my watch when the first mile beeped and saw 9:24. Now, I'm 24 seconds behind my bare minimum pace. I have to make that up. So, I push and push, but I just feel like my tank is empty. I just feel like this whole run today, getting up late, not doing my normal routine, has ruined everything. Maybe the lack of caffeine is playing into this. My legs are just slugs. Pure slugs. So sluggish, they won't respond to my brain. But really, my brain is sluggish, too. I'm not trying very hard. I want to. I really do. I want to be faster, but how can that happen if the brain and body don't care? So weird to not have control of things. I don't even feel like the same guy who ran yesterday. I'm going to have to realize that preparation is important. Go to bed early, don't eat junk, quit eating an hour before bedtime, get your rest, wake up on time, do your routine. This sucks right now. Some pebbles have found their way into both my shoes. They are wedged to the side and below my feet So, that's great. A deer fly bites my left shoulder and I just want to scream out and cry. But I don't. I just run a little bit faster. The second mile is 9 minutes even. So, I didn't make my time deficit worse, but no improvement either. Still 24 seconds behind bare minimum. And now this running is starting to drag. Why am I doing this? This really isn't fun right now. Lots of problems today, all coming to a head now. I see a few turkeys down Pee Lane. I have to kinda go pee, but I think I'll hold it. I don't want to stop, since it will take time I don't have to lose. Also, I don't want to go down that trail with those turkeys around. It would probably be my luck, today of all days, that turkey would attack me in my vulnerable state. So, I just run by. No time, don't think about it, just run. A bunny is alongside the road. I've passed it several times now, and it doesn't care. It moves its ears a bit, but just lazily munches on the clover and stuff. It doesn't seem to be very bothered about anything. I wish I was that bunny right now, just not a care in the world. The fourth and fifth miles are exactly the same pace, and I've now climbed my way back into a positive pace position. I'm just under 9 min/mile, and only five minutes to go to 50. And that's when I realize, at my current pace, there is no way in the world I can get to 5.65 miles, which is my lowest distance output this month. After all the trouble today and the false starts and failings and stress and everything weighing on my mind and shoulders, I don't think I can also take having the worst distance day ever. So, I speed up. I don't know where it comes from, I don't know how I turned it on. I don't know if I can keep it up, but it is only 5 minutes. Less than 5 now. Just give it all you got. Breathe in and out, move those legs. I start to run with my arms now. My legs are done and not very good right now. No pain, just dog tired. My arms, though, I pump and pump. They will force my legs to move with them. Pump, pump, breathe, let's go.

This is it. I glance at my watch a dozen times. Getting closer. I have no idea of my pace, I just see the time getting closer to 50 and my distance slowly inching up. 5.30, then 5.45. Come on, no time left, let's do it. Just as the timer changes to 50:00, my distance turns over to 5.65. I couldn't make this stuff up. So, I don't earn the awful recognition of worst run day today. I tied my worst, but a tie is a tie. My pace on that last mile was 7:59. I don't know where it came from or how I got it out of me, but thank goodness. The running is over, but now I have to get moving. Shower time and get to work. Hurry up.

POST-RUN: Well, I'm happy the run is over. I am not happy with the ultimate resulting distance, but I am happy with my final effort over that last five minutes to get to 5.65 miles. I have a headache now, which could be from the stress and not drinking coffee like normal. So, that'll be just great the rest of the morning. My weight after a shower was 167.2 pounds (down 0.1).

Wednesday, July 12 from 3:17 PM to 4:07 PM

Splits	Time	Cumulative Time	Distance
1	7:52.5	07:52	1.00
2	7:43.7	15:36	1.00
3	9:35.6	25:12	1.00
4	10:12.4	35:24	1.00
5	8:53.6	44:18	1.00
6	5:43.4	50:01	0.67
Summary	50:01	50:01	5.67 mi
Average Pace 8:49 min/mi			

PRE-RUN: There was a big thunderstorm with rain at 5:30 AM. It woke me up. I realized there was no way I was going to be able to run this morning like normal, because the ground was soaked and everything was muddy. So, I postponed my 50 minute run until the afternoon to let the ground dry. In hindsight, this was a mistake, but I'm not sure there was really any better alternative. I knew it was hot. I knew it was humid. I was not prepared for this. I wore my blue shorts and blue t-shirt and ball cap. Sunscreen all over. I stretched my legs inside my house and went out into the oven.

RUNNING: The first two miles were actually okay. Somehow, some way, I was able to get a really good pace going and was under 8 minutes per mile both times. And then I hit some kind of wall. You have no idea. I have no idea what happened. It was like someone hit a light switch and all my energy and ambition and fortitude disappeared. Once that beeper went off for Mile 2, showing a great pace, my mind quit, my body quit, and I became a zombie. As I slowed to a crawl, my body just wouldn't go forward. At 2.33 miles, I had to stop and walk. I was beaten down. The sun, the heat, the humidity, it was too much. I had to stop and walk. It sucked. I didn't know if I could get going again, but after about a tenth of a mile, I started to jog. My wife was out riding bike on the loop. She saw me and offered to go get my water bottle. If she hadn't been there, I'm not sure I would have been able to continue and finish the 50 minutes. As she went in the house, I went around the loop. I tried to wipe off the back of my neck, and felt over five bug lumps. I looked at my hand, and there were black gnats or flies or something stuck there. All sweat suckers, I guess. I looked in my arm hair, and they were there, too. I wiped my face with my hands, and same thing. Black gnats or something on my skin. It was pretty nasty. The sun went behind the clouds twice during that 50 minutes. Once at 1.42 miles and once at 4.33 miles. Those were important events, since it allowed me to catch a mental break and relieve the pressure of finishing this run under duress. Once in a while, the wind would blow, just enough to get a breeze across my legs, arms, and face. It was hot wind, but still better than nothing. Early in the run, a deer fly bit me behind my right ear. Later in the run, another deer fly bit me in the exact same spot. It must have been attracted to the wound or blood.

The second bite hurt more than the first. It made me angry. During mile 4, at the highway turnaround, my old friend the kestrel was perched high up on a power pole and chirping away. He looked right at me. Probably wondering what I was doing and why. I was just glad he didn't swoop down and peck my eyes out. That would have just been par for the course today. Dozens of times, around the loop, I had to shut my eyes while running. Either from exhaustion, bugs flying into my eyeballs (yes, it is as bad as it sounds), or trying to squeeze out the sweat and sunscreen. This run was one of the most uncomfortable I've had in memory. I couldn't get enough air, never enough air, and the air I sucked in was hot like a torch. The sun on my neck felt like a hair curling iron burning my skin. My wet clothes were suffocating me like a heavy blanket. I imagined that I was wearing a winter jacket and a heating pad was draped over my face. The temperature was 83 degrees with 70% humidity. That doesn't even sound that bad, but it must have been a perfect situation. Everything lined up to destroy my psyche and energy and ambition. At 3.24 miles, I stopped running to drink my water bottle. I walked and drank at the same time. I drank about 12 ounces of water. It was cold, but barely refreshed me. My stomach sloshed. I ran on. It slowly brought me back to life. About one mile later, the water was sitting low in my stomach and I wondered if it was a mistake to drink so much. The pressure stayed for a while but eventually I was able to ignore it. After mile 3 and 4, especially mile 4's 10:13 pace, I was resigned to having the worst distance for sure. Then, with whatever little mental power I had left, I decided that maybe, just maybe, my good paces from miles 1 and 2 could cancel out miles 3 and 4. Maybe, somehow, even though I'm on death's door, I can salvage this run. I immediately was determined to get at least 5.65 miles or bust. I looked at my watch, and saw exactly 11 minutes left. I was at 4.35 miles. Could I run for 11 minutes and get 1.3 miles? After all I put up with today? All the struggle, all the heat? So uncomfortable. Bugs everywhere. Sweat dripping, legs dead. Could I do it? I was about to find out. I noticed the brim of my baseball cap, which sticks out probably three inches from my forehead was steadily dripping sweat to the ground. My gosh, my hat is so soaked it's dripping sweat form the brim; I didn't know what to think of that. I pushed myself. I pumped my arms. I felt if I could somehow get mile 5 under a 9 minute pace, then I would have a chance to save this run. I needed to give myself a chance. Run, you stupid idiot, run. Come on. I stopped breathing multiple times for many steps. It felt better to not breathe. The movement of my chest, up and down, in and out, was uncomfortable in the heat. My exhaustion was maxed. It was just easier to not breathe sometimes, it is tough to describe it. But I ran on. My shirt was useless from mile 3 on. I had to wipe sweat with my dirty hands. I took off my hat many times to randomly swat over both shoulders to temporarily get the bugs to move away. Run, come on, move those legs. Let's go. You are so close to done, don't quit. Do you really want to look back at this run and see failure? What if you don't get an average 9 minute pace in this 50 minutes? What if this is the only run this whole month that you fail? Won't you hate yourself for that? Run, just run. Mile 5 beeped at a 8:53 pace. That gave me pause and a shot of hope. Screw you sun, screw you everything and everyone, I'm going to get this. Only five minutes left of this torture. Let's go. *She said where'd you want to go? How much you want to risk? I'm not looking for somebody with some superhuman gifts.* Yes, getting close. At 48:40, I had .15 miles to go to get to 5.65. I dug deep, it is so close, just a little more, pick up the pace, run hard, it is almost over. So close, almost over. Let's go. And 50 minutes was up. Somehow, I made it. I finished with 5.67 miles. It wasn't my worst distance yet. I beat it by .02 miles, not much, but it was enough. I had persevered. I was spent.

POST-RUN: I walked to my driveway, and it wasn't in a straight line. I couldn't keep a straight line for a bit and almost lost my balance. I kept squeezing my eyes shut to get the sweat and sunscreen out of them. I still couldn't use my shirt for any wiping. I really had to catch my breath. I swatted away the bugs that refused to leave me. I drank the last bit of water in my water bottle. I slowly bent over to start stretching my toes. Once my face was below my waist, the sweat beads shot off my nose and hat like machine guns and pelted the blacktop. The bugs were still bad and wouldn't leave me alone. They were landing on my exposed cheek and nose as I stretched my quads. One stung my neck again. This was really a bad day. Nothing was in my favor (well, except my wife. Without her, I couldn't have finished. I know that now. She saved me today.) Somehow I managed 5.67 miles, but it was not easy, it was not pretty, it was not fun. I need to get inside and drink some water and take a cold, cold shower. Maybe I'll drink the water in the shower? Boy, those first two miles really saved me. I have no idea how I got that pace. I guess I started out way too fast for conditions, which contributed to hitting the wall and basically stopping me from doing much of anything. But I did it. My weight after a shower was 164.4 pounds (down 2.8).

Thursday, July 13 from 6:22 AM to 7:12 AM

Splits	Time	Cumulative Time	Distance
1	8:36.9	08:36	1.00
2	8:20.6	16:57	1.00
3	8:22.7	25:20	1.00
4	8:26.0	33:46	1.00
5	8:20.9	42:07	1.00
6	7:31.0	49:38	1.00
7	0:23.1	50:01	0.06
Summary	50:01	50:01	6.06 mi
Average Pace 8:16 min/mi			

PRE-RUN: I woke up today at 5:30 AM, determined to put yesterday's debacle behind me. I did not want a repeat performance. I needed to take control and make sure I was ready for the run. It was cloudy outside, no sun visible, and the temperature was in the low 50s. I decided to wear Batman pajama pants, blue t-shirt, and ball cap only. No sunscreen. I was still tired from yesterday's draining run. I felt a little groggy, but a cup of coffee perked me up. Today is the 13th run in a row, but only about 13 hours or so since yesterday's run. So, that's not a whole lot of recovery time. But I really wanted to run in the morning, before it got too hot, and still give myself enough time to get to work. I stretched inside like normal. Today's routine was going as planned.

RUNNING: Once outside, I immediately noticed the cold air. It was way colder than I thought. The computer said it was about 54 degrees and 100% humidity, so I assumed it would still be hot or at least warm. Boy was I wrong. Two days in a row, the weather completely throws me for a loop. It was freezing outside. I was only wearing a t-shirt and pajama pants. I would have welcomed my black hood and long sleeve shirt, but I needed to get moving to finish the run in time and also to get warmer. And the wind was strong. Which made it even worse. Maybe the temperature alone would have been just fine. But the wind made it seem so much colder. It is interesting that the temperature went down 30 degrees but the humidity went up 30%. I started to run and the wind blew goosebumps all over my arms. If yesterday was running in a furnace, then today is running in a freezer. Only in Wisconsin can this happen. Two completely different days back to back. I can handle the cold wind on my arms and face, but it is pure pain when the wind blows hard in my ears. It is constant and uncomfortable. I concentrated on running and moving and tried to forget about the cold and wind. The entire sky was clouds, just light gray clouds. No sun anywhere. Body status check: I actually felt okay, for the most part, which surprised me. I thought my weariness from yesterday would continue today, but I actually didn't feel that tired during this run. The first mile pace wasn't bad, happy to see it around 8:36. My neighborhood buddy, the kestrel, flew around in the air, doing some long, lazy loops, barely flapping his wings. I guess he was riding the wind. I heard him chirp a few times, and then he disappeared. No neighbors outside. No dogs outside. No turkeys. And, thankfully, no bugs. I guess that is one positive from cold and wind. My right hip twanged a bit, and kept up a little pain for a few steps, but then settled down again. Mile 2 beeped and another good pace at 8:20. I remembered that 8:20 pace will get me 6 miles in 50 minutes, so I decided to keep it up and keep it steady. Don't change or fall behind, keep this going. Pump your arms. Think nice warm thoughts. You're already past 16 minutes, only 34 minutes to go. Ha-ha, only 34 minutes left in this freezer. Lucky you. I didn't bother to look at my current mile pace on my watch. I only glanced at my total time and miles a few times. I felt like I was running well enough, and every mile that would beep gave me a good indication of where I was at. Mile 3 pace ended up at 8:22, which is still good and consistent. Stick close to the 8:20 zone and this day will be fine. Keep up this pace. Remember your ultimate goal. You want that new half-marathon PR. Just imagine if you could keep up this pace of 8:20-ish the entire half-marathon on July 31st, don't you think you'd feel like a king. No need to go faster today, this is great, you need another day under your belt, you need another no-injury day. Just get this good and get it done. Don't worry about the weather anymore. Suddenly, a streak of pain went down my left neck from jaw bone to breast bone. It was there and gone in less than a second. I don't know what that was. Maybe a big nerve got triggered? I was just running like normal, so I'm not sure what it could be. I don't think that has ever happened to me before. I hope it doesn't happen again. First I saw the kestrel earlier, and now I see a huge harrier hawk flying over my head. It is gray and white, maybe some tan, but it is tough to focus on it as I run. He does a fast wide loop in the air and heads back to the woods. Two flying carnivores today, nothing much else around. Miles 4 and 5 are more of the same. I kept up a good pace. In mile 4, I went a little slower, it was my worst mile, but still within 6 seconds of the 8:20 goal. At 42 minutes, I see that I have 1.05 miles left to 6 miles. I do a quick calculation, which in my tired state takes a bit longer than normal. I need to get under 8 minutes on this last mile. Time to pucker up buttercup. You can do this. Start picking up those feet and pumping those arms. Get your breathing under control and slow. Focus and concentrate. I felt like I had a little bit of a kick left, so I started to run faster. I really wanted it. It was going to be close once again. It seems like I've been in similar positions before. I continued to ignore the wind and cold the best I could, but running faster just augmented the wind. My ears were screaming for warmth and quiet. Just get this done. Mile 6 beeped at 7:31 pace. I did it. Just over 6 miles at 6.06. Once again, I got something I ran hard for. Those little victories will keep adding up. You cannot get a best distance mileage every day, but take these daily victories for what they are. They are a test of your mettle. You did good. Nice kick at the end. You had some fuel in the tank. You kicked in the afterburner. Now, get inside. Get warm.

POST-RUN: Overall, I'm happy today. I finished with just over 6 miles. That will help to get my daily average mileage up. The last mile was a sprint, but it wasn't so bad. No significant new injuries popped up. Nothing got worse. Sure, I froze my butt off, but another 50-minute run is done. Thirteen down, 18 to go. My weight after a shower was 164.2 pounds (down 0.2).

Friday, July 14 from 6:30 AM to 7:20 AM

Splits	Time	Cumulative Time	Distance
1	8:39.0	08:39	1.00
2	8:34.5	17:14	1.00
3	8:35.5	25:49	1.00
4	8:37.3	34:26	1.00
5	8:26.4	42:53	1.00
6	7:08.0	50:01	0.96
Summary	50:01	50:01	5.96 mi
Average Pace 8:24 min/mi			

PRE-RUN: I woke up to darkness. It was after 5 AM, but the sun was nowhere to be found. It is sad to see the days start to get shorter and shorter. It feels like just a few weeks ago it was light out by 5 AM and didn't get dark until after 9 PM. Now, that's all changing and the days are shrinking. I can't believe how fast this year is flying by. *These are the days to remember, because they will not last forever. These are the days, cuz time is gonna change, you've given me the best of you. Now I need the rest of you.* The air felt cool by the open window, so I decided to wear extra clothing today. I put on my Batman pajama pants and two shirts, one short sleeve and one long sleeve over the top, along with my black hood and ball cap. I had one cup of coffee and did my morning stretches. My stomach was off and on yucky. I think I may have eaten too much food last night with double cheeseburgers and onion rings. I had stomach pains last night before bed, too.

But, at this moment, everything seemed fine, so I was ready to go out and get it. I decided to run another consistent race again, no need to kill myself. I still need to run 17 more days after this, with the half-marathon PR prize looming. Keep your focus on that.

RUNNING: I took off determined to just do a natural run. Don't push it and don't wimp out. Just keep it calm and consistent. All I need to do is finish another 50-minute run. You aren't going for any records. Just before the first mile beeped, my stomach was doing some little gymnastics. It felt a little roily and bubbly, but after about ten seconds, that either went away or I didn't notice it anymore. The first mile was 8:36, not bad, not great, just right in the middle. Good enough. No sun at all. And miraculously, no bugs. That's probably the best part. Good combo with no sun and no bugs. The wind was very slight, and the coolness wasn't bad. I was glad I wore my extra layers of clothes, and so far, my black hood wasn't giving me any issues. I had left hip pain during mile 2. That lasted just for a bit, and maybe it worked its way out. I could hear the neighborhood kestrel chirping like crazy at my neighbor's house. I'm glad he is over there, because his constant noise has become annoying. I hope he moves on soon. We called the local DNR guy and he said he is aware of the fledgling kestrels in the area. Apparently other people have called to complain. He said they will move on eventually, after they learn how to take better care of themselves, or if their parents move to better hunting grounds. I hope that is soon, because this kestrel has either gotten too friendly or too brazen. I'm literally just waiting for when it attacks me. It has already flown right near different windows in our home and hovered while squawking and looking menacing. Mile 3 beeps at 8:35 pace. Again, so far very consistent. All in the 8:30s. Not gonna be anything special, but just fine with this. Running around the southwestern curve of the loop, I got a sudden shooting pain in my left part of my chest. It didn't last long, but I wonder what caused it. I immediately stretch out my arms in front and back and up and down and out, seeing if maybe my arms needed some better circulation. They did seem heavy, and the stretching and moving them out of a normal running motion did them some good. At this point, about halfway done with my 50 minutes, I noticed I really stunk bad. This long-sleeved shirt I'm wearing has been in use for many, many months. It is always washed, of course, just like all my clothes after any exercise, but I think sweat and stink has permeated itself into the fabric. It might be held together more with stink than threads, for all I know. It is basically falling apart, with so many holes opened up around the neck line and shoulders. But it feels comfortable and familiar which is why I wear it. But, I realize it might be time to retire it and toss it in the garbage. Just too stinky. During mile 4, my left knee twinges a bit, both in front and back. I just kinda ignore and forget about it. It went away at some point, but I don't remember when. So, about 4.5 miles done, and I am very happy with my consistent pace. I've done what I set out to do. Keep running and finish this. I look at my watch and see I have about 9 minutes left and I'm at 4.78 miles done. I ask myself if I have anything left in the tank to get to 6 miles in 9 minutes? *But she said where you want to go? How much you want to risk? I'm not looking for somebody with some superhuman gifts.* I say I'm going to try, let's go for it. So, I pick up the pace and start to run hard. My eyes only glance at the watch a few times in the next few minutes, but as time is running out and I'm still not at 6 miles, I catch myself glancing many more times. It is going to be close. I gave it my all, especially at the end when that last .96 miles was at a 7:26 pace or faster. But I couldn't catch it. I ended up with 5.96 miles. I had shot for 1.22 miles in 9 minutes, but only got 1.16. I think I only needed about 10 or 15 more seconds, and I would have had it. So close, yet so far away. Again, this just proves the point on how important pace is and being consistent and how a few seconds here, a few seconds there, can really add up and ruin the ending. Over those first 4.5 miles, could I have gone 10 seconds faster? Sure, but I didn't realize at the time how important that was. If I could do it over, I would have run slightly faster. And I know what pace I need to get 6 miles in 50 minutes. It is exactly 8:20 pace, and I knew I was over that every time my watch beeped at each mile. I just let it go.

I'll have to try to continue to run and be consistent, but get closer to that 8:20 area so the kick at the end can still catch the 6 miles. I walk back to my driveway, but I have to close my eyes and take some good, deep breaths with my face pointed at the sky. I am winded after that last sprint.

POST-RUN: I am happy that Mother Nature finally threw me a softball. The weather was good, the bugs did not bother me, and my body felt good overall. I completed the 50-minute run without any real issues. And I was able to sprint at the end, which shows I still have the ability to kick it when needed. I did my waist bend to touch my toes and my back cracked twice. That felt good as it must have been compressed from all the running. My weight after a shower was 164.4 pounds (up 0.2).

Saturday, July 15 from 7:44 AM to 8:34 AM

Splits	Time	Cumulative Time	Distance
1	8:05.0	08:05	1.00
2	7:55.5	16:00	1.00
3	8:07.4	24:08	1.00
4	8:15.4	32:23	1.00
5	8:26.6	40:50	1.00
6	8:10.0	49:00	1.00
7	1:01.2	50:01	0.13
Summary	50:01	50:01	6.13 mi
Average Pace 8:10 min/mi			

PRE-RUN: I slept in a little later today, because it is the weekend. I felt pretty good overall. I drank a cup of coffee and did my stretches. I wore my green ninja turtle pants, blue t-shirt, ballcap, and lots of sunscreen. It looked sunny and windy outside. No clouds in the sky.

RUNNING: I took a bunch of deep breaths. I wasn't really looking forward to running today. I think the amounts of runs I've done are taking a toll on me, both physically and mentally. I feel like I'm fighting a war on two fronts, and I'm not sure if I can hold out. Today is day 15. I have 16 more to go. I start off okay, and the first mile is uneventful. I feel pretty good, a little tired, but nothing too bad. I get a pebble in my right shoe at mile 1.32. It stays there, moving around for the remainder of the 50 minutes. It was bothersome but not awful. Should I have

94

stopped to take it out? Maybe, but then I always worry about the jarring stoppage and trying to restart a run. Not only physically getting my body moving again, but the mental strain of firing the engine back up and getting motivated for the uncomfortable future. I decided not to stop and just deal with it. My left hip flared up a few times, and pretty much just lowly rumbled in the background, popping up once in a while to say hi and stick a fork in some flesh or tendon. I finally saw a small bunny today. It was standing next to one of the big ones that I see just about every day. The baby was very cute and fluffy. I yelled at it to say hi and how cute it was, but it didn't respond other than to jump into the weeds. I guess it doesn't like strangers. The sun stayed out and stayed strong the full 50 minutes. Not one cloud to break it up. The wind helped a little, especially out on the highway turnaround, where the wind can fly down the highway, and is like a refreshing cool bath. But as the run went on, I lost all energy and enthusiasm again. My mile paces were good, but they were hard to attain. I could feel each mile slipping away, with me going a little slower. And it was getting harder every mile just to get the pace that was slower than the previous one. I started to doubt myself. How could I finish a half-marathon? I need to do it in 16 days. I can barely think about finishing this 6-miler. I feel all spent and this isn't fun right now. Where'd my enthusiasm go? How come it disappears? I have to stay mentally tough. Just get through this one more day. I wonder how endurance runners can do what they do. It is mind-boggling to me that they can run 50 to 100 miles at a time. Do they have unique body parts or chemicals or proteins? How do their legs and feet and minds last that long? I think I'd be nothing but a quivering stump if I tried anything like that. No bugs today, well I should say there were a few that buzzed by me, but no attacks, no successful landings, no bites. The loop is in pretty bad shape again. There are more tractor tire tracks everywhere, thanks to my neighbor Tractor Man. As the miles slowly went by, I felt like I would get over 6 miles for sure. But it wasn't easy by any means. At 45 minutes done, I was still at 5.5 miles. With 2.5 minutes left, I only had .21 to go, so I knew I had it at that point as long as I didn't fall down or stop. I ended up with 6.13 miles, which is my 3rd best distance this month. The whole run though was problematic. I just felt completely uncomfortable and unfocused. It was hard to breathe, and I kept using my mouth way more than my nose to breathe. My running cadence and stride felt off, too. I tried to adjust while running, but gave up, never really sure if I was improving anything or making it worse. Lots of self-doubt today. Even at the end, I'm seriously unsure if I'll be able to complete a half-marathon.

POST-RUN: In my driveway, I did my post run stretches. My back cracked twice. I found out I have a small blister on my right foot, on the left side of my big toe. It is just a white bubble right now. It'll burst soon and provide me another reminder of why running is not glamorous. I had to suck in lots of big air after the run. I just couldn't catch my breath or get to a point where I felt normal again. I need to reevaluate things to make sure I'm still setting myself up for success. I think I really, really need to follow my rule of not eating after 8:00 PM anymore. I keep breaking that rule. Also, I need to drink more water during the day and get more sleep. Also, I really think running early in the morning is the way to go. Even starting the extra hour later today messed me up. It just adds that much more heat and sun and humidity. Fifteen days done. Sixteen days to go. Keep your mind in the game. You can do this. My weight after a shower was 164.0 pounds (down 0.4).

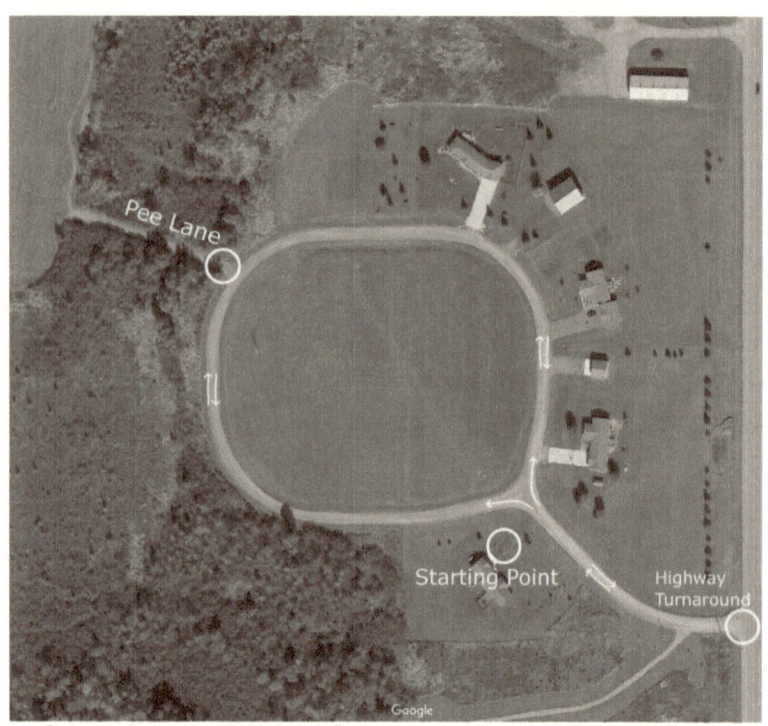

This is my running loop with noted locations.

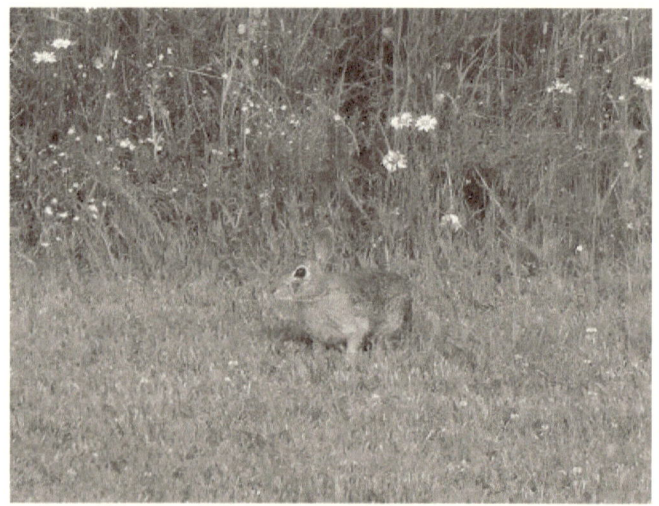

A familiar rabbit I would see many times.

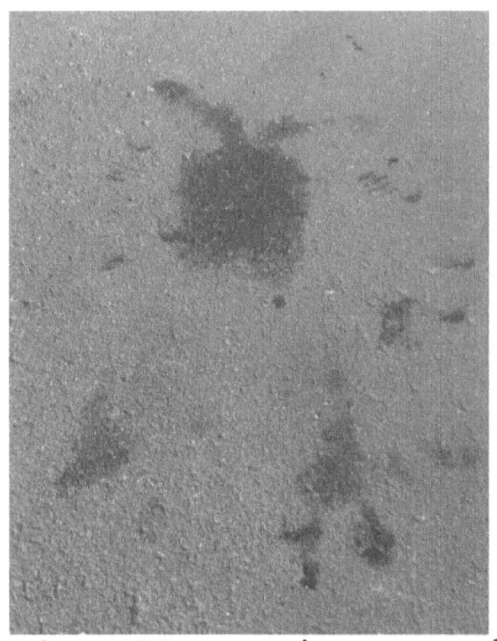

One of my Sweat Man creations on my driveway.

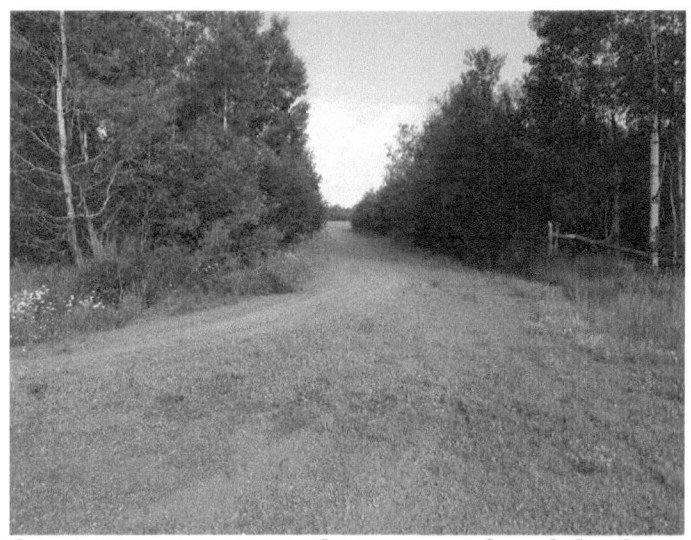

This is Pee Lane on the west side of the loop.

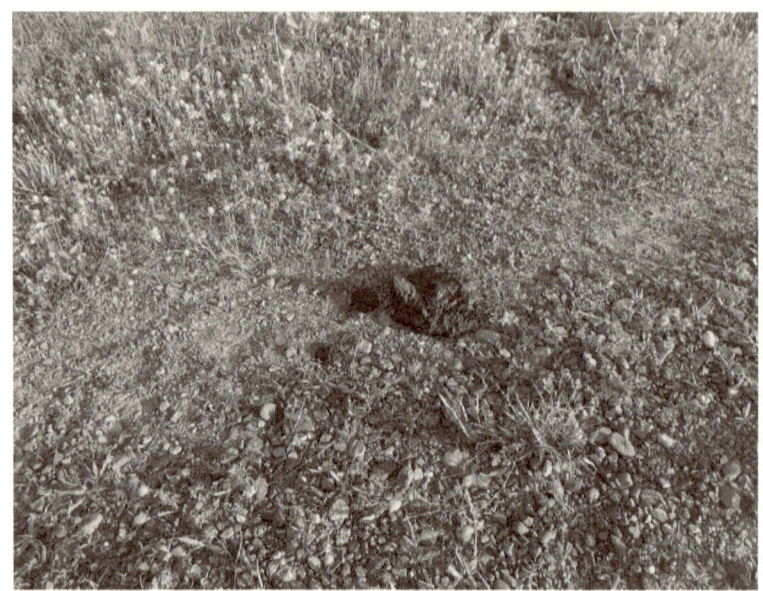

A big bear plop that I ran by for many weeks.

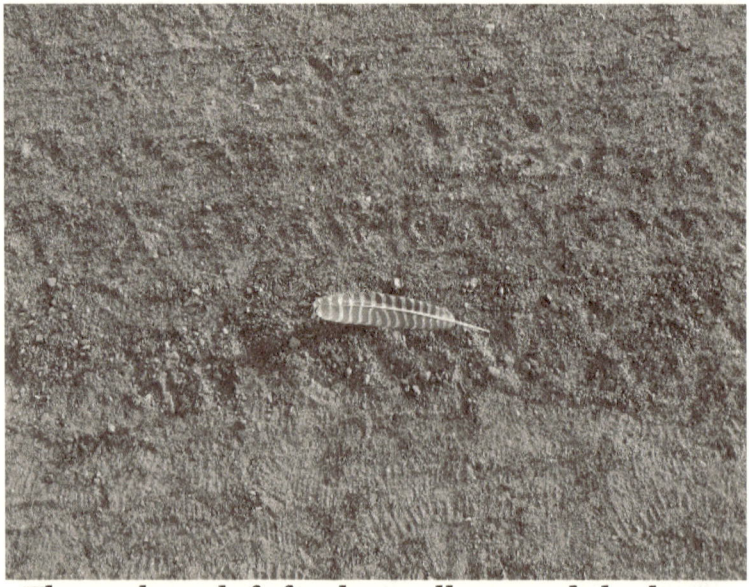

The turkeys left feathers all around the loop.

Sunday, July 16 from 6:55 AM to 7:45 AM

Splits	Time	Cumulative Time	Distance
1	8:09.6	08:09	1.00
2	7:49.3	15:59	1.00
3	7:43.3	23:42	1.00
4	7:45.0	31:27	1.00
5	7:42.0	39:09	1.00
6	7:31.3	46:40	1.00
7	3:20.0	50:00	0.47
Summary	50:00	50:00	6.47 mi
Average Pace 7:44 min/mi			

PRE-RUN: I woke up determined to get outside before the weather had a chance to rev up and kill me. I worried about my left Achilles heel, not sure if it will last this whole month of running. It is twinging and twanging all the time now, not just during stretches, but normal walking, too. I guess it isn't all the time, but enough that I've noticed it. I've heard about runners blowing out their Achilles tendon, and it doesn't sound fun. I think that tendon is important for many things, you know, like standing upright, for instance. So, then, just as quickly as a blink, I decide to just screw it. I think, who cares. Maybe instead of worrying about all this stuff and injuries and running technique and times and distances and run-on sentences, just run, period. Maybe go out there with a calm attitude. Smooth and easy. That became my new mental mantra. Smooth and easy, easy and smooth. I read about that in the Born to Run book. I'm about halfway through the book. The White Horse guy said it. I'm going to start doing it. Smooth and easy. I wore sunscreen, blue shorts, blue shirt, and ball cap.

RUNNING: The run started off with a bang. Literally. I had just run down the little leg of the loop to the highway turnaround and a gunshot blasted without warning. It sounded like nearby, just past a small woods, and it scared the dickens out of me. My shoulders scrunched, my head darted around, and I ran away quickly. For a millisecond, I wondered if the bullet would hit me. I heard the sad or angry squawking of many sand hill cranes coming from the woods area. I don't know if they were the gunshot target or if they were close enough to be alarmed. I only heard one gunshot, though. The loop was in decent condition. I saw huge tractor tracks, but instead of having deep treads that rip up the dirt and rocks, these treads were flat and helped to smooth it all out. So, you know the famous saying, what one tractor taketh away, another tractor giveth. Or something like that. Anyway, easy and smooth. I lived it. I ran it. Smooth and easy. My arms were swinging. I didn't control their speed. My legs were running. I didn't control their speed. I didn't care about my foot strike or hip pain or breathing. I just ran. I noticed that my running stride became quick and choppy. Instead of long strides and graceful running, my feet were quickly turning over. Chop, chop, chop. I just went with it. The very next highway turnaround, a black pickup truck just passed by and I ran out into the highway for a bigger turning curve, and the strangest thing happened. The very second I was in the truck's wake, the air suddenly became warmer, the wind stopped, sounds stopped, and it was like I was running in a vacuum. For that split second, I was all alone in the world and nothing was there. Then, out of the truck's wake and back on the loop, everything went back to normal. Was that an out-of-body experience or just a middle-aged man's deteriorating mind? Inquiring minds want to know. I only looked at my Garmin watch, maybe, ten times this entire run. I looked when the miles beeped and then at the end of the run to make sure I stopped the watch at 50 minutes. Otherwise, I ran without worrying about it. Most of this 50-minute run is a blur. I just moved around the loop, going about my business. The temperature was good, the wind was refreshing, and no bugs bothered me while running. My left hip pain was there, but I ignored it. Or embraced it. Not sure exactly. It was there, I was there, and that's all. I didn't control my breathing. When I paid attention, it seemed to be nice and slow, not scared breathing or short, quick, I might die breaths. Of course, maybe just by paying attention to my breathing, I automatically change it. Like those photons in quantum entanglement that I'm hearing about in the news. Just by observing them, you change them. So, maybe when my mind clicks over to my breathing channel in my head, my breathing changes to normal. As the miles go by, and I'm still feeling good (I like this easy and smooth idea) I remember that I ate horribly last night. We got home late from a family thing, and instead of just drinking some water or something, I decided to eat two large pieces of pizza and a bottle of root beer at 10:30 PM. Why? Why? I don't know why. Because I'm an idiot, and I even thought about how I shouldn't be doing this while I was eating it. That's the opposite of self-control, but somehow, I'm not seeing any negative consequences on the loop today. Everything is easy and smooth. Oh, and my earworm song loop is gone. I don't think I heard any song lyrics in my head during the entire run, which I appreciate since I was getting sick of them. The fledgling kestrel is at it again, flying around, screeching and chirping, looking for food. It flutters away from tree to tree in my front yard as I get closer on the loop. I remember when my back hurt so bad at work, this was like 3 or 4 years ago, that I would need to lie on the floor and just close my eyes. I guess all the years of sitting at work, bad posture, and whatever finally made my back give out. That was years ago, and that was why I started long distance running. Course, back then, a long distance was half a mile, then a mile. And my pace was like 10 to 12 minutes, and it was hard. I'm glad I've stuck with it. My back pain is gone now. Mile 6 beeps on my watch, but I didn't look down at that one. I don't know why, maybe I forgot. I just kept running, and then 20 seconds later, I looked at how much time I had left. I just kept going, easy and smooth, until the 50 minutes was over. I stopped running. My watch said I had a new 10K PR of 47m 53s. My most recent 10K PR was only like 9 or 10 days ago, so I couldn't even remember what it was to compare them. Did I beat it by a few seconds or a minute? I was thinking maybe 30 seconds. I was on the far side of the loop from my house, so I had a built-in recovery walk to get home. I wasn't breathing hard. I felt good all over. I actually smiled. Maybe I was happy for a bit. Either today was an aberration, or there really is something to this easy and smooth mantra. I'll do it again tomorrow. You know, I was just thinking, no one told you how to run as a kid. You just ran. You didn't care about technique or foot strikes or strides or correct arm and head placement, breathing. You just ran like a kid. Maybe that's what I did today. I just let my body decide how to run for itself.

POST-RUN: So, wow, I'm not sure what to say. I can't explain this one very well. I basically started the run with the mindset of not caring. I didn't care how my body felt or if I was hurt or if I was running the right way or if I was going too fast or too slow. I just ran. I kept telling myself to run easy and smooth, smooth and easy. Let your freewheeling mind determine the correct combination of the million different body variables. I did not consciously try for this 10K PR, but I guess all that smooth and easy action added up to shaving 26 seconds off my previous best. My weight after a shower was 164.6 pounds (up 0.6).

Monday, July 17 from 6:37 AM to 7:27 AM

Splits	Time	Cumulative Time	Distance
1	9:13.2	09:13	1.00
2	8:34.4	17:48	1.00
3	8:40.3	26:28	1.00
4	8:35.9	35:04	1.00
5	8:26.3	43:30	1.00
6	6:30.8	50:01	0.84
Summary	50:01	50:01	5.84 mi
Average Pace 8:34 min/mi			

PRE-RUN: I woke up sore in both hips. My left hip was worse, so I did my regular morning stretches and gingerly walked around the house. I had no idea what I would be able to do today on my 50-minute run. Could I even get going? I wasn't positive, and that was a little scary. Plus, my left Achilles tendon continued to twang-twang like 90% of the time. I went outside in Mario pajama pants, red t-shirt, ballcap, and lots of sunscreen.

RUNNING: I was late getting outside, so everything felt like a rush. Looking at my watch, I would barely have enough time to do the run, shower, and shoot out the door to work. And the prospect of running with pain didn't terrify me, it just scared me a bit. The prospect of doing long term damage terrified me, though. I didn't want to get injured so close to my goal. I pressed go on my watch and took many gentle steps down the first part of the gravel road. I was testing out my hips. They didn't feel smooth. But they also didn't feel like I was making things worse, so I decided to keep going. Just on a whim, I decided to change my running mechanics. Instead of pounding my left heel I tried to run with more of my forefoot hitting the ground. Almost like a sprinting movement, but not that fast. It almost made my left hip feel better, but that could have just been my mind making it so. At this point, I really couldn't tell reality from my wants. I wanted this new running technique to fix everything. I wanted it to be the answer. And where did I get this idea? From that book I'm reading called Born to Run. Now I'm in the chapter where barefoot running is discussed and it is making a lot of sense. I don't want to run without shoes, but maybe I can run and pretend. Like it says in the book, if you run without shoes, you do not heel strike. If you do, you quit running because you are going to bloody your heel and destroy yourself. Runners without shoes run on the front of their feet, so that's what I was going to imitate today. Mile 1 was slow at a 9:13 pace. I had to do better than that if I didn't want this whole run to be worthless. It took me many laps to feel my way through how running like this should feel. It felt a little alien. I used to sprint in high school, so I ran on my foot balls then and it felt fine and normal. But now today, doing this similar stride but going much slower felt strange. Almost like I was running in place. But I made progress. And my left hip didn't hurt any worse. My right hip pain went away. I finished the second mile and then the third mile at good paces. I was just happy to be still running and not on the ground in pain. At times, it felt like my legs were a sewing machine needle, going up and down, up and down, almost too fast to feel normal. The constant sound of my feet hitting the dirt and gravel reminded me of Bob Ross painting on a canvas. With his wide brush, he would kinda stab at the canvas to create trees or shrubs. That "shush, shush" noise is what I heard now as I ran. My far side neighbor's old dog was outside behind his fence, so he barked as I ran by. I hadn't seen that dog out in a long time, so it was okay. When mile 5 beeped, I wanted to end this run with a roar, not a whimper, so I started to speed up. I noticed that speeding up was very easy using this stride, since my feet were already in racing form, if that makes sense. My old technique with the left heel strike would require that I first have to speed up before I could switch to running on the balls of my feet. With this different technique, I'm already on the balls of my feet, so it was just a matter of going faster. I finished with 5.84 miles, which is just fine with me. I wasn't positive I'd even be able to finish, so I'm happy. Also, I guess we'll see how I feel the rest of today and tonight, to see if anything is better or worse. I do feel my left lower calf is sore now, which I'm guessing is due to the change in technique.

POST-RUN: I finished the whole 50 minutes while trying a new stride. I do not know what to think. My left hip pain didn't get worse, my right hip pain went away, but now my left lower calf muscle is sore. I could see two Sweat Man stains on my driveway, so I stepped to the left and created number 3 with my post-run stretches. My weight after a shower was 165.6 pounds (up 1.0).

Tuesday, July 18 from 6:40 AM to 7:30 AM

Splits	Time	Cumulative Time	Distance
1	8:14.6	08:14	1.00
2	8:10.0	16:25	1.00
3	8:03.9	24:29	1.00
4	8:10.3	32.39	1.00
5	8:20.5	40:59	1.00
6	8:12.6	49:12	1.00
7	0:49.2	50:01	0.11
Summary	50:01	50:01	6.11 mi
Average Pace 8:11 min/mi			

PRE-RUN: Woke up kinda late again. I stretched and drank one cup of coffee. My left leg is a hurting unit. Both hip and lower calf were telling me to beware their wrath. I wore blue shorts, gray t-shirt, ballcap, and sunscreen.

RUNNING: It was very humid outside. My shirt soaked all the way through and by mile 4, I had no clean or dry spot left to wipe off my face. The heat wasn't bad, but the humidity was. There was a slight wind to help cool off. A few bugs kept buzzing by my ears. A few successfully landed right by my earhole. That is so annoying. I did my forefoot striking the entire time. It wasn't effortless. It wasn't smooth and easy today. My goal is to run without pain and have fun, but today was not that day. I had to check myself many times to make sure my back was straight, my feet were hitting underneath my body, and my arms were moving well. My breathing was okay, not too stressed or forced. I don't think I over-exerted myself that way today. My left hip hurt, but it sort of went away during the run. I don't remember when, maybe mile 4. My lower left calf was unhappy the whole time. It didn't get worse but for sure didn't get better. And after mile 4, I felt a blister on the bottom of my left foot right by the base of the big toe. And my right foot, just the whole forefoot, felt raw and sore. I felt it every step. At mile 5.32, a big turkey flushed out of the weeds by the road as I was running by and he ran ahead of me around the curve. It was pretty funny, because he stayed on the loop at a good trot about 30 feet ahead of me. He ran that way for almost a fifth of a mile. I smiled and laughed. That felt good. I am happy with my overall distance and pace and everything. My pace was very consistent for every mile, an average of 8:11 min/mile. My aerobic activity was fine today, now I just have to get my physical parts healthy again. I had no problem breathing today. Never got uncomfortable in my chest or throat.

POST-RUN: My previous Sweat Man stains were gone from the blacktop driveway, but I made a whopper of one today. My shirt was very soaked. It looked soaked, it felt soaked, and it was heavy. I stretched my calf muscles a little extra and will probably do it more throughout the day. I'll have to watch that blister on the bottom of my left foot. I guess my whole left leg is a litany of trouble. Hip, calf, and foot. My weight after a shower was 164.0 pounds (down 1.6).

Wednesday, July 19 from 6:13 AM to 7:03 AM

Splits	Time	Cumulative Time	Distance
1	9:08.8	09:08	1.00
2	8:47.8	17:57	1.00
3	8:45.5	26:42	1.00
4	8:43.4	35:26	1.00
5	8:18.8	43:44	1.00
6	6:16.7	50:01	0.79
Summary	50:01	50:01	5.79 mi
Average Pace 8:38 min/mi			

PRE-RUN: My calf muscles are sore again today. I woke up earlier today to hopefully get outside faster. Last night around 8 PM, I ran an easy mile with my son around the loop. He was wearing Crocs. That was fun to be with him, taking it pretty nice and easy. It is very foggy outside. I decided to just wear my green turtles pajama pants, blue t-shirt, and ball cap. No sunscreen, since the fog was so thick. I had one cup of coffee and did my stretches.

RUNNING: I felt sluggish and pitiful the whole run. I just had no energy to get going. My form felt wrong, but I stayed with it. Running on my forefeet for 50 minutes. The fog was really thick. It lasted for about 4 miles, and then the sun came out. The fog was gone, and I didn't have sunscreen on. So, for about 20 minutes I ran from one tree's shadow to the next around the loop, whenever it was available. One funny thing, about mile 1.32, a turkey burst out of the weeds and ran down the loop. Very reminiscent of the other day when I chased a turkey. This was even better because I could just barely make the turkey out through the fog as he ran away, and it was very ghostlike. Very Stephen King's "The Mist"-like. My forearm hair was full of dewy drops from the fog or humidity. They were pretty. My hip pain didn't show up, which is good, but the inside groin area of my left leg started to twinge. I'm not sure if that is just something new or because of my new forefoot strike technique. I don't like the idea of that groin tendon becoming injured. I think I'll have to watch some running videos on YouTube or something to get some more tips and ideas. The garbage truck monster showed up in the fog. He was hidden at the end of my neighbor's driveway but made all the clang, clang noises possible, and I heard his low grumble before coming upon him. I turned around in a weird spot and went the other way. I didn't want to end up on some TV show about strange deaths. Yeah, this guy who runs every morning knew the garbage truck was there in the fog, but he decided to run behind it anyway. What did he think was going to happen? It ran him over. Also, with this same thought in mind, I never got close to the highway turnaround. I always heard cars or trucks but could not see them. I didn't want to take any chances, so I turned about twenty feet earlier than normal. I kept my breathing good and steady. I thought I did a good job of that, but maybe that was because I wasn't pushing too hard. I'm not sure. It's not like the run was easy, but with a pace of 8:38, it wasn't hard either. I think the dreary weather and my new running technique combined to give me a bad day.

POST-RUN: I'm really questioning myself now if this technique of forefoot striking is correct. With 2 days of it under my belt, it doesn't seem better. I don't want to go back to heel striking, but there must be a good compromise. I feel like I'm running on my tippy toes. And my blisters are getting worse and my calf muscles hurt more. My weight after a shower was 164.2 pounds (up 0.2).

Thursday, July 20 from 6:19 AM to 7:09 AM

Splits	Time	Cumulative Time	Distance
1	9:01.6	09:01	1.00
2	8:53.0	17:55	1.00
3	8:59.9	26:54	1.00
4	8:53.8	35:48	1.00
5	7:45.6	43:34	1.00
6	6:26.9	50:01	0.84
Summary	50:01	50:01	5.84 mi
Average Pace 8:34 min/mi			

PRE-RUN: I woke up not excited to test out my gimpy calf muscles. They were still extremely sore from the last two days of running like a sprinter for 50 minutes. I wore green pajama pants, blue t-shirt, ball cap, and lots of sunscreen. There was fog outside again, but not as much as yesterday morning, and the sun looked like it was here to stay. I had one cup of coffee and did my normal morning stretches.

RUNNING: It was nice weather. A little foggy, little sunny, not too hot, not too cool. I gave up on running with my tippy toes/sprinter technique/forefoot thing. I decided just to run the way I had been before. And my hip pain came back a little, but mostly it is the inside left groin area that was bothering me. On my first journey around the loop, right before Pee Lane, there was a huge pile of green-brown poop steaming in the early sunshine. It looked like a horseshoe crab or maybe a trilobite. I looked around quickly trying to see if the perpetrator was still around. I'm guessing either a bear or a sasquatch. I really hope it was a squatch. I think I chased the same turkey from yesterday again. This time, there wasn't as much fog, but the same thing happened. I'm running around a curve and out pops a turkey and it runs away from me down the loop. Just like we were in a race. This time I actually put on the jets and gave chase. The turkey was too far away for me to catch, plus he was fast. Every time his foot hit the ground, little poofs of dirt appeared and dissipated. I wish I had that turkey's speed. Of course, the turkey slowed down and turned into Pee Lane. Maybe they assume I won't follow them there. Maybe one of these next times, I'll throw him a curveball and suddenly change course and chase him down Pee Lane. After mile 4, I only had about 14 minutes left. I knew my average pace was pretty poor and very close to or over 9 minutes per mile, which I am determined to always beat. I didn't want to have this run be my worst ever, so I gave it all I had. I ran fast, but still kept my old technique. Every time I noticed my left heel strike, I tried to correct it. It's not perfect, but maybe I'll get better over time. I really pushed it and ended mile 5 under 8 minutes, and finished with 5.84 miles. On my last lap around the western curve, the kestrel was perched high up in a dead tree. The highest branch, cheeping and chirping. When I looked him in the face, and he looked back in my face, he quit chirping. For a few seconds anyway. Once I ran past, it was noisy again.

POST-RUN: I feel like I did awful this run, like I just couldn't get anything going. My pace at the end of 8:34 is misleading, since I really had to run hard the last 14 minutes to even get that. The first four miles were dreadful. There were times I looked at my watch and saw paces of 9:34 and 9:12. I shouldn't be anywhere that slow at this point in my training. I only have 10 days left before I try for a PR half-marathon. And my left hip pain is back again. But my calf muscles weren't destroyed and actually feel better, I think. So, am I at a crossroads? Either do heel strike and face the wrath of hip and knee injuries, but calf muscles and blisters go away? Or do forefoot attack, but face the wrath of calf muscles and blisters, but hip pain goes away? Why can't I find a happy medium? Where is it? Not much time to find it, either. Twenty days down, 11 to go. My weight after a shower was 164.0 pounds (down 0.2).

Friday, July 21 from 6:35 AM to 7:25 AM

Splits	Time	Cumulative Time	Distance
1	8:38.5	08:38	1.00
2	8:21.5	17:00	1.00
3	8:24.2	25:24	1.00
4	8:57.3	34:22	1.00
5	8:55.0	43:16	1.00
6	6:44.6	50:01	0.79
Summary	50:01	50:01	5.79 mi
Average Pace 8:38 min/mi			

PRE-RUN: I ate too much junk last night. A huge double cheeseburger and package of mini donuts from the local fair. And a big turkey sandwich. And candy, good lord, the candy. What am I doing this to myself for? I woke up with zero energy. That doesn't bode well for the run. I wore blue shorts and t-shirt with black hood and ball cap. Looking outside, I saw lots of fog again, and it felt cold by the open window, so I decided to wear the hood. Had one cup of coffee and did my morning stretches. Took me awhile to get outside, just no urgency. My left groin tendon is tender. Otherwise, for the most part, I feel okay.

RUNNING: Temperature is good, little cool, feels good. I think black hood was the right decision, at least early on. My left groin tendon hurts with every left step. Is it from overuse? Did I pull it or wrench it on a previous run? Is it from changing my running form? The whole reason I tried different stuff was because my left hip was hurting on the outside. Now, my left hip doesn't hurt, but my groin does. Did I just trade one injury for another or are they the same thing? I just cannot get going. Again, I look at my pace on my watch and I see numbers above 9:00 minutes per mile. That is undoable. That can't happen. I feel like I'm moving fast enough to be below that. I know I'm not going super-fast, but still not as slow as 9:00 min/mile. The first few miles are okay, but my groin slowly gets worse as the miles add up. Not so bad that I'm limping or anything, but I can feel every step. Something is sore in there, and it does not like the running motion. I end up with 5.79 miles. Not very good, considering 5.65 is my low point. I sure hope this gets better soon. I need to eat better, too. And get more sleep.

POST-RUN: Stupid deer fly bit me in the hand while I was doing quad stretches, and some other bug buzzed inside my right ear. I don't know how to run anymore. I changed up my running form twice in the last five days, since nothing feels right and parts of my legs hurt. I've gone backwards. My left hip and/or left groin tendon and/or calf muscles and/or foot blisters hurt depending on how I run. At this point, I just need to keep myself together with duct tape if need be. Now that I think about it, I think my current downward spiral happened right after my July 16 run where I got my new 10K PR. All I know is this: I cannot get injured any worse or this month's goal will be in serious jeopardy. My weight after a shower was 164.0 pounds (no loss or gain).

Saturday, July 22 from 7:08 AM to 7:58 AM

Splits	Time	Cumulative Time	Distance
1	8:22.1	08:22	1.00
2	7:56.5	16:19	1.00
3	8:12.0	24:31	1.00
4	8:12.7	32:43	1.00
5	8:22.3	41:06	1.00
6	8:14.4	49:20	1.00
7	0:40.7	50:01	0.09
Summary	50:01	50:01	6.09 mi
Average Pace 8:13 min/mi			

PRE-RUN: Woke up and didn't move too fast. Waited until after 7:00 AM before going outside, letting the sun come up more. I was thinking maybe all the fog and general gray dreariness outside was bringing me down, so I wanted the sun on my face. Overall, I felt pretty good. My left hip and left groin tendon were not painful, and when I stretched, they did not pull or feel bad. That gave me some hope and confidence. I had one cup of coffee. I wore my green pajama pants, gray t-shirt, ballcap, and sunscreen. I just remembered I had a dream last night about a bear that chased me around the loop. It didn't feel like a very long dream, and I don't think the bear caught me. But, it was scary.

RUNNING: I didn't really think about much today during the whole run. Or, at least not much topical variety. It was mainly controlling my breathing and focusing on my legs and feet. I tried to adjust my foot strike every once in a while, so that I didn't heel strike the entire 50 minutes. The first mile felt too slow, even though I ended up with a good time of 8:22. But there were times I looked at the watch, and it was over 9 minutes per mile. The second mile was great at 7:56. I really didn't want to push it, and I'm not sure if I could have even if I wanted to. I didn't have a whole lot of gas in the tank today. I had enough to just go out and do what I did. I don't think I could have run faster. I was really hoping not to make my left hip injury or left groin tendon any worse. And for most of the 50 minutes, I either didn't have pain or couldn't feel the pain. So, that was nice. Speaking of pain, around mile 5, I felt a sharp sting in my right forearm. I was positive a deer fly had got me, but when I looked down, it was the tiniest little black fly. I am not sure how that little thing could produce such a painful bite. Nevertheless, it didn't take much to put an end to that. I tied my shoelaces a little tighter today, hoping that would help with controlling my blisters. Try to stop the rubbing. I think that worked, but maybe it was a little too tight, because I could feel my feet pushing against the top of the shoes with every step. Just a slight annoyance. Other than that little black bug, there was a weird sound by my right ear. It slowly built up and I was wondering what that was. I put my finger in my ear, but nothing there. Then I felt behind my ear and some kind of fly was back there. It flew off, but I wonder what it was doing back there. Didn't bite me, but just making some strange "digging around" sound. No buzzing.

POST-RUN: Okay, I'm fairly happy with today's run. My overall pace was 8:13 minutes per mile, which is just fine for day 22. I didn't have a lot of extra energy, but I did have enough to keep going today. I didn't get hurt any worse, and basically finished the day without any major pain. So, that is a win-win. Maybe I'm on my way to healing. During my post-run stretches on the blacktop, I laid down right next to a horror show. An earthworm was dead and there were dozens and dozens of little ants devouring it. The ants must have thought they hit the jackpot. Twenty-two days down, 9 to go. I just need to hold out and not make any big injury mistakes before my day 31 showdown with Mr. Half-Marathon. I think I can, I think I can. My weight after a shower was 164.0 pounds (no loss or gain).

Sunday, July 23 from 6:37 AM to 7:27 AM

Splits	Time	Cumulative Time	Distance
1	8:52.1	08:52	1.00
2	8:39.0	17:31	1.00
3	8:45.9	26:17	1.00
4	9:07.0	35:24	1.00
5	8:44.5	44:09	1.00
6	5:53.0	50:02	0.70
Summary	50:02	50:02	5.70 mi
Average Pace 8:47 min/mi			

PRE-RUN: Woke up with a little bit of hip pain and lower back pain. Other than that, everything else felt good. I wore blue shorts, red t-shirt, and ball cap with sunscreen. I had one cup of coffee and did my morning stretches. Oh, and my left Achilles tendon, for like the last 2 weeks, is twinging. When I stretch it, it snaps together and twangs like a guitar string.

RUNNING: My left hip/groin area hurt the entire time. It wasn't awful pain but still annoying and worrying. Still no energy today. I finished, but not without concern for the half-marathon coming up in 8 days. I just don't know if I'll be able to finish the half at this point. It is pretty sad to come this far and then either not be able to finish and/or not get the PR I'm going for. I really need about 2 or 3 rest days to heal up and revitalize my body and mind. But that wasn't part of my stupid plan and changing the plan now or not running every single day would make me feel like a failure. During mile 1 today, I looked at my watch and saw paces about 9 minutes per mile. It is so demoralizing to see that, because I feel like I'm trying hard, and I don't know if I can give any more oomph to get going. Runs that felt easy and smooth with good paces just a few weeks ago are getting hard to come by. I sang Bon Jovi's *Shot Through the Heart* a bunch of times around the loop. I tried to concentrate on my breathing and ignore my left hip/groin pain. A couple deer flies bit me on the back during mile 3. Mile 4 was not pretty and my pace showed it. Not impressive at all, and might be a harbinger of things to come if I can't shore up my weaknesses and store up some energy. The half-marathon PR pace I'm shooting for is less than 8:51 minutes per mile. Mile 1 and mile 4 today were worse than that. I can't have that during my half-marathon try. It just won't work. I'm going to need every mile under that pace to have a chance, because I don't know how I'm going to finish that race. At this point, I don't think I will be able to finish it as strong as I want to. I really had to push again today to finish mile 5 and part of mile 6 to get the 5.70 miles. That's gotta be like one of my top 5 worst distances. Nothing to be proud of.

POST-RUN: Stupid deer fly bit me in my right calf muscle when I was doing my left quad stretch. That was an awkward situation where I had to bring my right foot up to my butt and twist around on my belly and punch the bug with my right fist. My weight after a shower was 164.0 pounds again (no loss or gain).

Monday, July 24 from 6:26 AM to 7:16 AM

Splits	Time	Cumulative Time	Distance
1	9:17.9	09:17	1.00
2	8:22.5	17:40	1.00
3	8:35.6	26:16	1.00
4	8:42.6	34:59	1.00
5	8:35.1	43:34	1.00
6	6:27.4	50:01	0.83
Summary	50:01	50:01	5.83 mi
Average Pace 8:35 min/mi			

PRE-RUN: I've read that some runners don't even stretch before running, and they have experienced fewer injuries. I'm still not sure about that, but today I did much less stretching before going outside, just to try it out. I drank one cup of coffee and wore my red pajama pants and gray t-shirt. It felt cold outside by my window, so I wore my black hood and ball cap. No sunscreen, as there was a thick soup of clouds in the sky.

RUNNING: Once outside, I didn't bother with my extra stretches. I just took a deep breath and clicked go on my watch. It was chilly outside, that's for sure. No sun at all. Just gray clouds everywhere. A little bit of fog around the loop, but not much. Just dreary. At one point during the first mile, when I felt I was going nice and smooth and injury-free, I looked at my pace and saw 9:36. I was surprised how slow I was going. I tried to get going, but short of all-out sprinting, I didn't want to make a huge move. So, mile 1 ended with a whimper and a 9:17 pace. Then, something happened. Mile 2 started on a decline on the opposite side of the loop from my house and I just started going faster. And it felt fine, too. Nothing really hurt. I felt like I was standing taller, running faster, running more efficiently, and things felt great. I immediately thought about why I couldn't run this way all the time. I was able to keep it up for the most part and mile 2 ended with a good pace of 8:22. Miles 3 to 5 were all about just keeping a nice steady run going. I wasn't trying to do anything other than finish respectably and injury-free. I paid attention to my breathing and my feet, but mostly thought about the half-marathon and making sure I have everything ready for it. I'll probably have my kids keep an eye on me and bring water when needed, and maybe my wife and older kids would be willing to ride bike beside me for part or all of the race. I realize it's only one week away. Seven short days and I'll be running for my PR. I ended with 5.83 miles today. I'm feeling pretty good, and I'm ready for tomorrow. Let's start knocking these out. Twenty-four days down, 7 to go.

POST-RUN: After that first awful mile, I settled into a good pace for the rest of the 50-minute run. The great news today is the injury report. Nothing new and nothing got worse. In fact, knock on wood, my left hip/groin area felt much better than yesterday.

Both during and after the race. My weight after a shower was 164.2 pounds (up 0.2).

Tuesday, July 25 from 6:28 AM to 7:18 AM

Splits	Time	Cumulative Time	Distance
1	8:40.9	08:41	1.00
2	8:37.1	17:18	1.00
3	8:43.3	26:01	1.00
4	8:42.0	34:43	1.00
5	8:41.6	43:25	1.00
6	6:36.4	50:01	0.81
Summary	50:01	50:01	5.81 mi
Average Pace 8:37 min/mi			

PRE-RUN: It was cloudy again this morning, with just a hint of showers coming down. I decided to wear blue shorts and gray t-shirt and black hood, in case of cold. No need for sunscreen as the clouds were super thick with no sun shining through. Again, today I tried very little stretching. I'm hoping that is the super-secret key to healing from my injuries. I've read about that before, but I just don't know if it's true. There seem to be so many different conflicting ideas in running. Just read any magazine from month to month. Just when it seems like "this" is what you need to do, someone says nope, do "this" instead. So, anyway, I just did some quick back cracks and hamstring stretches. I had one cup of coffee and needed to hurry to get this 50-minute run in before going to work.

RUNNING: No extra stretches outside either. Grass was wet. I try to take exaggerated, high steps to keep my shoes dry. It doesn't work that well. No rain at the start. I clicked go on my watch and started moving. My first 10 to 20 steps are always gentle and probing. I want to make sure that I don't get a sharp, unexpected pain. I never know if they will feel good or bad. But today, those first few steps felt fine. So, away I go. I am determined to run a good, solid, consistent pace today. Not super-fast, just fast enough to beat my half-marathon PR. I know that if I run every mile below 8:51 pace, I will get my PR. Mile 1 beeps, and it felt good. I breathed well and my hip pain is gone. Good pace of 8:40. In mile 2, it starts to sprinkle again. And it doesn't let up. Kinda fun to run in the rain. I was lucky there was no thunder or lightning, because I would hate to have to stop. Safety first, of course. This is one of those rare rain days. I've been pretty lucky this whole month. But running in the rain can be kinda neat. It is not a hard or heavy rain, just a light soaking, and so it is easy to run in. I think I remember reading somewhere that you'll get wetter if you move in the rain by walking or running than if you would just stand in place. Well, I'm not going to test out that theory today. Today, I just need to run and run well. Easy and smooth, keep it going. Mile 2 and mile 3 are great. Good on target. I think that if I can just bottle up this feeling and this pace, then that half-marathon PR is as good as mine. Now, I'm not a complete idiot. I know that what I'm doing this month is probably not the right way to train for everybody. Heck, I don't even know if it will work for me. Running every single day for 50 minutes, and only getting close to 6 miles is not the best way to train for a 110 minute run and 13.1 miles. But, for some reason, I think this will work. Time will tell. Only 6 days left in this month. Miles 4 and 5 are almost identical. It is still raining. Not hard, though. No bugs or animals out. As I run around the loop, I've also given up on exclusively running in the middle of the lane and have floated to either edge of inner or outer. I don't know why. I'm just letting my body choose. I think I was trying to control too many things like how to run, where to run, how to breathe, what to concentrate on. At some point a few days ago, after I had a bad run and it was hard and I didn't know what I was doing anymore, I just said screw it. Run like you want to run. Who cares if it isn't what the experts say is right. If it feels right to your body, just do it. After mile 5, I looked at my watch and saw about 5 minutes to go. That's when I kicked it in a little bit, trying to make sure I get at least 5.65 miles. I could noticeably feel my speed increase, and it didn't hurt. I didn't get winded, but I could feel the extra breathing necessary to produce the speed. Ended up with 5.81 miles. Not bad. Not bad at all. Twenty-five days down, 6 to go.

POST-RUN: Well, today went great. I'm very happy with my consistent pace over all the miles. I didn't get hurt any worse, and there might be a chance that my hip and groin is improving. I could feel it once in a while, but the majority of the run felt good. My weight after a shower was 164.0 pounds (down 0.2). I guess I've plateaued on losing weight or this is some sort of sweet spot. I can pinch plenty of fat on my belly yet, so I think I'm just stuck in a rut. All the extra food I eat (and candy) probably isn't doing me any favors. Did I mention that I ate a large peanut butter sandwich and twin pack of nutty bars and 2 glasses of milk at 9:15 last night? And I'm trying to behave, honestly.

Wednesday, July 26 from 6:28 AM to 7:18 AM

Splits	Time	Cumulative Time	Distance
1	8:52.5	08:52	1.00
2	8:46.1	17:39	1.00
3	8:47.5	26:26	1.00
4	8:40.6	35:07	1.00
5	8:35.9	43:43	1.00
6	6:18.3	50:01	0.77
Summary	50:01	50:01	5.77 mi
Average Pace 8:40 min/mi			

PRE-RUN: I wore my red pajama pants and blue t-shirt outside and ball cap. It was sprinkling out again. No sun, just complete cloud cover. Funny, the first 24 days were almost all dry, and now two days in a row I have to run in this wet stuff. I was short on time, so I drank my coffee, and hurriedly went outside to get started. I also did an abbreviated routine of stretches.

RUNNING: The rain did not let up. It thundered about three or four times over the 50 minutes, but no lightning. And the rain never seemed like anything more than a light shower. No storms or anything. So, in a way, it was neat and refreshing. And in another way, it was annoying and soaked me through and through. My first mile was slow, I didn't want it in the 8:50s, but it is what it is. I tried to make sure the remaining miles were consistent but in the 8:40s or below. The gravel and dirt on the loop started to become moist and spongy. That didn't make for very good foot traction. It never got muddy, though. The humidity combined with the rain so I never had a clean face. I always felt like wiping it, but had nothing to wipe with. The sky was nothing but white and gray clouds. My body felt pretty good. I tried to curl my big toes right after taking a step to help stretch out my feet, but it isn't something I can do for very long. I think it helps, but who knows? Nothing really hurting, until about mile 3. I noticed my lower left knee in the front started to sting or twinge or whatever. I'm sure it is from overuse and all the running changes I've been doing. Again, today, I just ran like how I used to. After mile 5 beeped, I looked at my watch, and saw I only had a little over 6 minutes left. I knew I would get close to 6 miles, but I decided to run faster anyway. I for sure wanted to make sure I got over the 5.65 mile marker. I ended with 5.77, and by this time, the rain was really coming down. No longer a sprinkle. Not a direct downpour either, but really a good rain.

POST-RUN: I was soaked so I didn't bother to stay outside any longer. No stretches on the blacktop. I just walked right in the house. My weight after a shower was 162.8 pounds (down 1.2). That is my lowest yet.

Thursday, July 27 from 6:22 AM to 7:12 AM

Splits	Time	Cumulative Time	Distance
1	8:09.5	08:09	1.00
2	7:53.3	16:03	1.00
3	7:55.4	23:58	1.00
4	8:10.2	32:08	1.00
5	8:25.0	40:33	1.00
6	8:01.1	48:34	1.00
7	1:27.0	50:01	0.20
Summary	50:01	50:01	6.20 mi
Average Pace 8:04 min/mi			

PRE-RUN: I woke up at 5 AM. I did minimal stretches again. I had one cup of coffee and one small bar that my wife made. It was full of grains and vitamins and healthy stuff to give me strength, I think. It was kinda like a piece of tasty cube-shaped sand. I felt pretty good overall physically. My calf muscles must be healed up completely now. And my left hip felt better than it did yesterday. I wore my blue shorts, blue t-shirt, and ball cap. The sun was rising in the low sky, so I put on lots of sunscreen and headed outside.

RUNNING: The grass was completely wet. So, my shoes were nice and moist from the lawn before I even made it to my driveway to start my run. The sun was in full force, no cloud cover, so I'm glad I wore sunscreen. It was a light blue sky. Not one cloud anywhere. Very pretty. I clicked go on my watch and took off. The first few gentle steps reported no injuries or worries about my knees or hips, so I started to run with gusto. Two rabbits were out by the side of the loop in the grass. Man, they get big eyes when I run by. The loop dirt and gravel is slightly wet, too. I can feel the little pieces of dirt and pebbles kicking up and sticking on my legs and falling into my socks and shoes. I was thinking that I wanted to shoot for a pace of 8:30 minutes per mile. I figure if I can hit that every mile for the first 6 miles, then that'll put me in a good position to finish the half-marathon with enough gas in the tank. Ultimately, I just need to get an average pace faster than 8:51/mile to beat my PR. Mile 1 beeped at 8:09. That's just fine with me, and I wonder if that is too fast today. But then I remember that I've read that it might be smarter to run faster in the beginning miles and hold on until the end than run slower in the beginning and hope your kick in the end will catch up to what you want. So, I decide to stick with that speed, and maybe go a little faster. Somewhere in mile 2 I looked at my watch and my pace was 7:47, so that made me smile. That's about a minute faster than I've been doing the last few days with my slow consistent runs. I don't want to wear myself out here, of course, but it feels good to be running faster. I think I should keep running this fast to get my muscles to remember this effort. Remember this feeling, because the half-marathon is looming. Mile 2 beeps and it is a 7:53. Which is great. The pebbles and sand are piling up on my legs. I can look down and see my shoes kick them up and out and in and over and all around me as I run. My legs feel good. No pain, except just every once in a while, my left hip feels a little sharp. I hope that means it is mostly healed and not just one good pop away from exploding. Mile 3 is a great follow-up with a 7:55. Now we are cooking. I'm not breathing hard. I'm not in pain. I'm just in running mode. I'm tired, don't get me wrong. Well, I mean I'm using energy. I'm not exhausted or anything. But I feel comfortable running at this pace today. I think I should do this all again on half-marathon day. Just try to pound out as many miles as close to 8:00/mile pace as possible and hold on to the finish. But boy, I have no idea what the weather will be like. Or how I'll feel. That's why I wonder if I just shouldn't keep going today. You know the weather is decent. You are kicking butt on these first few miles. But it just doesn't feel right. I decide to just run the 50 minutes and stop again. I'm so close to the end of this month, no reason to mess it all up. *Who sent for me? You sent for me? Now this looks like a job for me, so everybody just follow me, cause we need a little controversy, but it feels so empty without me.* Eminem just burst into my head. That's a blast from the past. Haven't listened to him in a long time, but he has so many good songs. I should go back and listen again. Well, no matter what comes on half-marathon day, I'll just deal with it, I guess. I slowed down for miles 4 and 5. I didn't want to, but my muscles and energy were on auto-pilot and that's what I got. I saw about 7 turkeys down Pee Lane. They were way at the end. I wonder if they'll watch me on half-marathon day. No other neighbors or dogs out. Just me, myself, and Irene. I'm all alone, pounding out these miles. With 5 miles done, I see I have about 9 and a half minutes left on my watch, so I decide to kick it up and run harder. Try to get my body ready for more punishment. Mile 6 is a great 8:01 pace. Dirt and pebbles are flying everywhere as I run. I end up with exactly 6.20 miles when the 50 minutes is done. Not bad.

POST-RUN: Wow, I'm really happy with that run. I actually made it to 6.20 miles and didn't kill myself doing it. I definitely was running fast and hard that last 10 minutes, but nothing overboard. I actually thought about just keeping running to finish the darn half-marathon. But, I decided not to. I think I'm a little worried about it. I'm not sure if my body can hold up for another 50 minutes after the first 50 are done. And I haven't been training for that distance, so I'm worried I've put blinders on my body and muscles and they think they need to work hard for 6 miles or 50 minutes and then they are done. I wonder if it'll be a rude awakening on July 31st. It might end up being all mental after the first 50 minutes, if my body gives up. I took my shoes off and there was so much sand and dirt and gravel in there, I can't even tell you. I probably could have opened my own beach. How that all got in there and didn't hinder my running is beyond me. My weight after a shower was 161.6 pounds (down 1.2). That is now officially my lowest weight in 15 years.

Friday, July 28 from 6:44 AM to 7:34 AM

Splits	Time	Cumulative Time	Distance
1	8:33.2	08:33	1.00
2	8:25.3	16:58	1.00
3	8:33.3	25:32	1.00
4	8:35.3	34:07	1.00
5	8:33.8	42:41	1.00
6	7:20.1	50:01	0.88
Summary	50:01	50:01	5.88 mi
Average Pace 8:31 min/mi			

PRE-RUN: I stayed up too late last night reading part of Haruki Murakami's running book. It is interesting enough to keep me awake, and I didn't get to sleep until after 10 PM. So, of course, I slept in longer than I wanted. I didn't get out of bed until almost 6 AM. By that time, everything was a rush. A quick bunch of stretches, an abrupt cup of a coffee, and one sand-textured flavor cube that my wife baked. I wore my Batman pajama pants, blue t-shirt, sunscreen and ball cap. My left hip felt a little sore again.

RUNNING: It is very nice outside, no clouds, just the sun slowly rising in the east. Some nice shadows across the loop from bigger trees. I start my run and my legs don't feel too bad. But I can tell I'm still tired from my great run yesterday. There is a baby bunny in the grass alongside the loop. It is so funny to watch these guys tense up as I run by and they immediately form into a loaded rocket, ready to spring into the grass. They even make sure they point their entire body and head at the place in the grass they want to explode into. Then, if they don't think I'm a threat enough, they relax as I go past. But if I get too close, their eyes get huge, and those giant powerful legs send them shooting into the tall grass with one push. I decide to attempt a nice consistent run centered at about the 8:30 mile pace today. I figure that is still a fast time to help my body get ready for half-marathon day, but slow enough recovery from yesterday. About half way through mile 1, all the food I ate yesterday including 3 giant brats with fixings and nutty bars and cookies and ice cream come roaring back in my mind, and I wonder how I'm still alive. I treat myself so poorly. I know I have to do this 50-minute run every day. I know I need to get healthier to run the half-marathon, and yet every day I continue down a path of self-destruction. I do myself no favors eating like it is going out of style. That feeling of hatred and hopelessness lasts for a good twenty steps or so, but I soon go past it. I have to. If I dwell on it too much, I'll implode. I see those same big turkeys at the end of Pee Lane again. I'm guessing they live down there. That giant bear plop is still in the loop. I run by it every time and now I've decided to try to hurdle it each time. I try to time my footsteps to not stutter step. Sometimes I'm successful and hurdle it without messing up my stride. Other times, I have to throw my foot to the left or right just in time to miss stepping in it. So far, so good. No poop feet. My left hip is in pain. Imagine Dragons flows through the music center of my brain. *Pain, let this bowl of fire go through my brain, my god I can't complain, you've made me a, you've made me a believer. Pain!* Mile 1 and mile 2 beep, and I'm happy with what I've done. Right around the pace I want. I keep my breathing nice and slow. I don't need to punish myself. Just get through this run without getting hurt worse. Yes, your left hip is hurting, but it isn't going to ruin you. You can get through this. Keep up this consistent running, and get to recovery mode. Try to ignore the body. Look at the world. Look at what nature has given you today. A beautiful day. Full of sun and a nice breeze. You can float through this world. No one knows what you've been through, what you can endure, except for yourself. Keep pushing. Miles 3, 4, and 5 are very close in times. I'm doing a great job staying steady. At the highway turnaround, I see a guy in a truck I've seen the last few weeks. He and I always wave at each other. I have no idea who he is, but it is nice to be friendly. What do you have to lose to smile at someone? To be nice to someone? It might be the only time they get that pleasantry today. *Pain, you've made me a, you've made me a believer, believer. Pain.* I've got about 7 minutes left. So, keep running. Pick up the speed a bit, get going, get past the 5.65 mile mark. My left hip is screaming a bit, not every step, but it makes itself known. I try to run on my forefeet just to change up my stride a bit, maybe shift the pain. I think it works for a bit. I'm engaging different muscles, stressing different body parts, so I keep it up for another minute. Then, I change back to my normal stride and finish the 50 minutes with 5.88 miles. Not bad, quite happy with that.

POST-RUN: Well, I decided to run an 8:30 pace and that's exactly what I got. I don't think I've ever done that before. The odds must be pretty low to do that. Lady luck must be on my side today. Twenty-eight days down, 3 to go. I can do this, I know I can. A deer fly bites me in the neck below my chin as I walk to the house. Thanks. I owe you one. My weight after a shower was 162.4 pounds (up 0.8).

Saturday, July 29 from 7:00 AM to 7:50 AM

Splits	Time	Cumulative Time	Distance
1	9:01.8	09:02	1.00
2	8:50.2	17:52	1.00
3	8:55.2	26:47	1.00
4	8:46.7	35:34	1.00
5	8:46.1	44:20	1.00
6	5:41.6	50:02	0.68
Summary	50:02	50:02	5.68 mi
Average Pace 8:48 min/mi			

PRE-RUN: A gunshot rang out at 3:00 AM. It woke me up, of course. It seemed close, but when I looked out my bedroom window, I couldn't see anything strange. It was dark out and no obvious lights or source of the sound. I decided to try to sleep again. At 3:30 AM, 7 gunshots in a row, each coming about 3 to 5 seconds after each other destroyed the nighttime quiet. Now, I was awake. What was going on out there? Who in their right mind would be shooting a gun at this time of day? I hate you, I thought. Thankfully, that was the last of the gunshots. I finally went back to sleep, but woke up again at 6 AM and was up for the day. I drank one cup of coffee and did minimal stretches. I wore red pajama pants, gray t-shirt, sunscreen, and ball cap. My main mental goal today is not get hurt. Do not make anything worse. My hip is still gingerly stabbing once in a while. It needs to heal up in 2 days. So, today and tomorrow, those runs must be slow, recovery runs. You have nothing to prove today. Just to survive the half-marathon on the horizon.

RUNNING: I saw the same two or three bunnies alongside the loop again. They are pretty cute, and very fast. Sometimes, even though they are in the grass along the loop, and could easily jump into the tall grass and safety, they will jump out onto the loop, run down the loop in front of me about 10 or 20 feet, and then suddenly turn and dart into the grass. I wonder why they do that? My pace is pretty slow, I'd never have a chance to catch them anyway, even at my best. I'm well over 9 minutes per mile now as I look at my current pace, and I guess that's okay. I mean, I want it to be closer to 8:50, and I'll try for that, but this is okay for now. It does mentally hurt to run this slow, but I have to keep my brain on task and just finish this race. Because to run this slow also feels good. My hip isn't hurting right now. The goal is to finish without making my hip worse or adding any new injuries. This has to be a slow, recovery run. So, just suck it up and get it done. No reason to whine or worry or think you aren't doing the right thing. If you ran faster today, you would be doing the wrong thing. Duh! How are you even gonna start the half-marathon, let alone finish it, if you wear yourself out? Miles 2 through 5 are pretty uneventful. The sun is out. It is a nice temperature and I'm not sweating too much. I started this race a little late today, but I'm fine with that. It is the weekend. I'm kinda tackling this run and plan to tackle tomorrow's run with a laid-back attitude. Mile 5 beeps and I have about 5 minutes to go. Like yesterday, I pick up the pace so I don't get below 5.65 miles. I guess I set that minimum standard the very first day of July and I don't want to get below it. The 50 minutes is up, and I'm all sweaty now. I know I'll make a pretty good Sweat Man on my driveway. So, I do some quick stretches and kneel down. The front of my body, my arms, chest, legs, and shirt and pants, are all covered with little pieces of dirt and pebbles as I stretch my quads. I get up and the Sweat Man is there in all his glory. I use my hands and wipe off as much of the dirt and pebbles that I can. No need to go into the house with more of Mother Nature than I came out with.

POST-RUN: Well, I finished with 5.68 miles. That's about as slow as I can get and still not establish a new low. I'm happy with this run today. I don't feel any worse. Now, I just need to continue my day and not pig out on food. Just eat normal, healthy amounts and keep my energy level high. Twenty-nine days down, 2 to go. My weight after a shower was 164.4 pounds (up 2.0).

Sunday, July 30 from 7:08 AM to 7:58 AM

Splits	Time	Cumulative Time	Distance
1	8:35.1	08:35	1.00
2	9:05.0	17:40	1.00
3	9:10.6	26:51	1.00
4	8:56.6	35:47	1.00
5	8:35.3	44:23	1.00
6	5:38.4	50:01	0.66
Summary	50:01	50:01	5.66 mi
Average Pace 8:50 min/mi			

PRE-RUN: I wore my green turtle pajama pants and blue t-shirt, sunscreen, and ball cap. I drank one cup of coffee. Ate nothing else. I did my normal stretches today, nice and slow. I don't have much stress today. Just need to get outside, get it started, and end this thing. Last "warm-up" day before the big, main event.

RUNNING: I swallowed a bug. Lots of turkeys down Pee Lane today. All sunny, no clouds, just a few shadows on the loop since I started later. There is a pile of fresh green turds on the loop, looks like discarded wet green beans. During mile 1, I was hemming and hawing about whether to do my 50 minutes or just do the half-marathon today. It seems I've done that a lot, and I'm not sure why I keep thinking about it. I think it is probably because I'm scared that I might not do well on the actual half-marathon day, and I think if I'm doing well enough today, just keep going. But I keep coming back to the goal and promise I made myself at the beginning of the month (and continually through the month during my depressed days). Why change it up now, with one day left? Just do it tomorrow. No matter what happens, you will have followed your own plan. During mile 2, I somehow kicked up a rock which stabbed me in the right Achilles tendon. I have no idea how that happened. It kinda defies science and physics and life in general, doesn't it? How does my left or right shoe have the power to kick up a rock in the same direction I'm running and hit me square in the back of the right leg when my left leg is the one that is ahead of my right leg? I can't think about it too much; my brain will hurt. Other than my temporary right leg pain, my body is feeling good. My left hip and groin didn't give me any trouble today at the speed I was going. Miles 2 and 3 finish above a 9 minute pace, so I know I've made more work for myself than I wanted. Yes, I wanted to take it easy today, but this is perhaps coasting too much. I don't want to fall below 5.65 miles for the day, so for the next 2.5 miles, I have to speed up a little more than I wanted to. Instead of a consistent pace, I ended up doing something like a bell curve. In any event, I finished it. After 50 minutes, I got 5.66 miles and no injuries. That is a success.

POST-RUN: Only one day left. The day I have been working for. The day I hope I am ready for. I did enough today to finish the 50 minutes with more than 5.65 miles and not get hurt. I had to push a little faster than I wanted to during the last 5 minutes, but it is what it is. Come on, I got this. Just need to stay healthy and eat healthy the rest of the day. Get some good sleep. Wake up and dominate. It all comes down to this. Thirty days done. Thirty complete days of running 50 minutes each day. Only one day left. All that stands between me and the end of July is a half-marathon. I'm gunning for a new a PR, anything faster than 1hr 56m 01s. In the immortal words of Seinfeld's Izzy Mandelbaum, "It's go time." My weight after a shower was 164.2 pounds (down 0.2).

Monday, July 31 from 6:15 AM to 8:05 AM
(HALF-MARATHON DAY!)

Splits	Time	Cumulative Time	Distance
1	8:08.0	08:08	1.00
2	7:59.1	16:07	1.00
3	8:07.0	24:14	1.00
4	8:14.6	32:29	1.00
5	8:23.5	40:52	1.00
6	8:33.6	49:26	1.00
7	8:41.3	58:07	1.00
8	8:39.2	1:06:46	1.00
9	8:47.1	1:15:33	1.00
10	8:52.9	1:24:26	1.00
11	8:46.0	1:33:12	1.00
12	8:47.6	1:42:00	1.00
13	8:07.9	1:50:08	1.00
14	0:37.3	1:50:45	0.10
Summary	1:50:45	1:50:45	13.10 mi
Average Pace 8:27 min/mi			

PRE-RUN: If sleep is important, I am in some trouble. I woke up at midnight, 1 AM, 3 AM, 4 AM, and 5 AM. All because our wonderful neighbors are night bodies (i.e. idiots). I couldn't fall asleep right away after the car noise, loud talking, engine revving, dog barking, etc. has finally subsided. So, I'm not feeling my perkiest right now. I did my morning stretches and my left hip is not healed. It hurts when I stretch or move my hip a certain way. I'm gonna need to complete this run in pain, I fear. I have a water bottle, extra t-shirt, and extra ball cap at the end of my driveway. I'm wearing my blue shorts, gray t-shirt, ball cap, and sunscreen to start with. I'm listening to Imagine Dragons' *Believer* a few times to get psyched up. *Pain!* I hope the lyrics are embedding into my cells and subconsciously recorded somewhere in my gray matter. I'm gonna need a good mantra to finish this run. I take some deep breaths and just try to relax. I know I can do this. No time for doubts now. Just get out there and run how you know you can run. Thirty days of training has led to this point. Go get it. I do have a few butterflies in my stomach just for a second, but they flutter away. I'm okay.

RUNNING: I press go on my watch and blast off, determined to get as many fast miles under my belt as I can before my body knows what is happening. I keep my arms pumping and hear the mile 1, 2, and 3 beeps. They went by fast. Each time my watch beeps, I look down and smile. I'm so glad to see fast times. Right around the 8:00 minutes per mile pace is just great. This is starting out well. Now, just hang in there. Hold on and don't let go. I kept my breathing as steady as I could. I tried to stay focused but fast. Hook shot, hook shot, hook shot. Give it everything you got. I see many turkeys down at the end of Pee Lane, but none are out around the loop. So, I guess I won't have any impromptu teammates to run with today. I wore the same shirt for the entire run. I didn't think changing it would make that much difference and would only slow me down. I did not drink any water until after I was all done. That was just my choice, and I'm fine with that. The water bottle was right there at the end of the driveway. I passed it two dozen times, but I didn't get thirsty enough to go for it. I had to use the towel several times to wipe my face and neck and nose, though, because my shirt was useless after 6 miles. I changed my ball cap around mile 7, because it was so heavy from sweat. I was tired of seeing the drip, drip, drip of sweat falling off the brim right before my eyes. Right after I finished mile 6, my wife and son came out to ride bike with me for encouragement and to help me keep running my pace. Oddly enough, those miles they kept me company were also my slowest. I'm guessing that's just a coincidence, because at that point, I was slowing down anyway and my legs were getting tired. But I wonder what if anything would have changed if they weren't with me? I do know that I appreciate their company, because I can only think of so many things to think about before it feels like a severely broken record. My son talked to me about animals and video games and fishing and running. It was a good time. Even my youngest daughter got into the act, and she stayed in the driveway and handed me my towel and new ball cap when needed. Otherwise, she gave me air high-fives as I ran by, because when she gave me a real high-five the first time, she screamed out, "Eww, your hand is too sweaty." I think I repeated the Imagine Dragons'

Believer refrain about a hundred times. My feet felt good the whole race. My calf muscles felt good, my breathing was good, and my arms were moving well. In the later miles, when I was needing to concentrate more, I was forcing my arms to move with more power, driving body blows into the air. Take that! And that. Body blow, body blow, body blow. That helped to keep my legs pumping. The weather, I think, was perfect. It was cool when I started and the sun stayed behind a cloud for the first 4 or 5 miles. After that it was out, but it could have been much worse. Even so, I'm glad I started the run at 6:15 and didn't wait any longer. It would have just been hotter and sunnier. I don't think there was much of a wind, but again, with the cool, crisp air at 6:15, I was okay with that. Both my wife and son commented on how cold it was outside when they came out during mile 6, but I didn't feel that anymore. It was warm for me. My shirt was soaked, and it became a chore to try to wipe my face with it towards the end. Luckily, I had the towel available. At mile 9 was the first time that my pace went above 9:00 minutes per mile, so I think that is pretty good. Miles 10, 11, and 12 were just all mental. My body was tired. No doubt. I would have loved to stop, but my mind said no. I kept those legs chugging. I kept swinging my arms and picking up those feet. I kicked in everything I had left for mile 13, and that last half mile of the race, I ran as hard as I could. It felt like my left leg was flapping in the wind. My left hip was an un-oiled, creaky hinge hanging together with rust and spit. I was determined to keep running fast and consistent, smooth and easy, the entire race. I could tell I was gradually slowing down as the miles piled on, but I decided it was okay as long as I stayed under the 8:51 pace. I was glad I waited to run this race on the last day. I feel like I stuck to my original goal and accomplishing it makes it that much sweeter. All those 50-minute run days really made my lungs stronger and my endurance better. Even though jumping up from an average of 5.91 miles a day to 13.1 miles seems like a lot, my body was ready for it.

POST-RUN: I did it. I really did it. I'm very happy and relieved it is over. A great finish time, too. Wow, I was very relieved and excited to see my first 3 or 4 miles at or lower than an 8 minute pace. I figured I needed to start out fast and just hold on for the rest of the race, because toward the end, as I was slowing down, I don't think I could have sustained or increased myself to a faster pace for very long. Although, my kick at the end felt like I was flying. And my body was saying stop, but my mind was saying keep going. Not one mile got above 9 minute average pace, and only one mile was above the 8:51 pace I was trying to beat. At 50 minutes, I was right around 6.09 miles, so that made me feel like I was doing a good job. That beat my average 50 minute pace for the last 30 days, which was 5.91 miles. After the next 50 minutes, I was at 11.81 miles, which means I covered 5.71 miles in the 2nd 50. That is still above my worst distance of 5.65 from the past 30 days, so that is another win for me. In the end, I beat my PR by 5 minutes and 16 seconds. And my average pace was 8:27 per mile. That blows my previous 8:51 per mile out of the water. My lungs did not hurt at all during the entire run, and I wasn't breathing hard at the end. I walked a lot after finishing, just to let my body slow down and go back to normal. After walking and drinking water for many minutes, I did some nice slow stretches on the driveway and made my very last Sweat Man. It was a good one. Very wet. You'd be proud. Not one bug flew at me or bit me or landed on me this entire race. Isn't that strange? Now, I think I'm going to take a rest day tomorrow and be happy. Oh yeah, I was smiling during the last half of the race. I wasn't all the time, but I tried to do it when I thought of it. And I was smiling when my watch said 13.1 miles done and I had a new PR. I think if you can't smile when you are running or after you've run, then you're doing it wrong. Why go through the hours of work, the torture, the pain, the mental stress if you don't have fun doing it? I run for myself. I run for me. I'm just a regular person doing regular things. But this accomplishment today feels extra special. I cannot believe this month is now all over. I did it. I feel good about myself. My weight after a shower was 162.0 pounds (down 2.2).

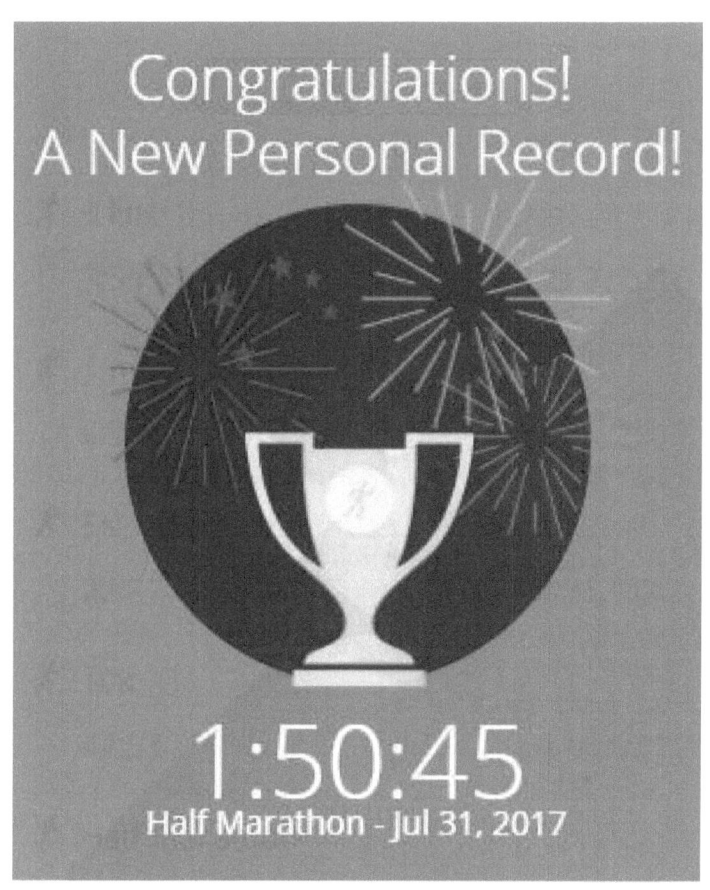

Final July 2017 Running Stats

Runs: 31
Total Distance: 190.31 miles
Total Time: 26h 51m 15s
Avg. Distance (50 min runs): 5.91 miles
Best Distance (50 min runs): 6.47 miles (Day 16)
Worst Distance (50 min runs): 5.65 (Day 1/Day 11)
Total Calories: 26,165
Avg. Speed: 7.1 mph
Avg. Pace: 8:28 min/mile

Now I can add July to my monthly mileage chart.

Month	Runs	Mileage	Total/Goal	Progress
January	6	30.32	30.32/60	-29.68
February	9	30.05	60.37/120	-59.63
March	14	40.83	101.20/180	-78.80
April	14	60.13	161.33/240	-78.67
May	30	100.61	261.94/300	-38.06
June	30	128.97	390.91/360	+30.91
July	31	190.31	581.22/420	+161.22

I have a healthy mileage buffer going into the last five months of the year. I feel pretty good about my chances of meeting my goal of 720 miles in one year. But, anything can happen with fall and winter looming. Five months is roughly 150 days. That's a lot of time for Mother Nature to devise obstacles for me. Perhaps deer flies with "frickin' laser beams attached to their heads" or something?

Author's Note

Thank you for reading about my 31 days of fun and pain. I had a blast putting this all together. I hope you enjoyed it.

Less than two weeks after I got my half-marathon PR, I also gutted my way to a new 5K PR. So, for the 2017 year, I've bested all my PRs in the 1 Mile, 5K, 10K, and half-marathon distances. I hope to improve myself for many years to come.

You can read more about my running stats, successes, and failures on my blog. Let me know what you think and leave a book review on Amazon.

Manley Peterson
August 2017

manleypeterson.blogspot.com
Twitter @ManleyP23

www.ingramcontent.com/pod-product-compliance
Lightning Source LLC
Chambersburg PA
CBHW050449290526
45786CB00006B/2222